MW00905784

The Familiar Stranger
Who Lives In Our Home

THE FAMILIAR STRANGER WHO LIVES IN OUR HOME

Dealing with Alzheimer's Every Day

Robert J. Betterton

Author of *The Compliant, Curious And Critical Catholic*

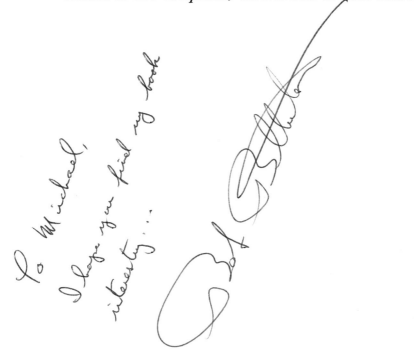

iUniverse, Inc.

New York Bloomington Shanghai

The Familiar Stranger Who Lives In Our Home
Dealing with Alzheimer's Every Day

Copyright © 2008 by Robert J. Betterton

All rights reserved. No part of this book may be used or reproduced by any means, graphic, electronic, or mechanical, including photocopying, recording, taping or by any information storage retrieval system without the written permission of the publisher except in the case of brief quotations embodied in critical articles and reviews.

iUniverse books may be ordered through booksellers or by contacting:

iUniverse
1663 Liberty Drive
Bloomington, IN 47403
www.iuniverse.com
1-800-Authors (1-800-288-4677)

Because of the dynamic nature of the Internet, any Web addresses or links contained in this book may have changed since publication and may no longer be valid.

The information, ideas, and suggestions in this book are not intended as a substitute for professional advice. Before following any suggestions contained in this book, you should consult your personal physician or mental health professional. Neither the author nor the publisher shall be liable or responsible for any loss or damage allegedly arising as a consequence of your use or application of any information or suggestions in this book.

ISBN: 978-0-595-49075-2 (pbk)
ISBN: 978-0-595-60959-8 (ebk)

Printed in the United States of America

To Mona,
Who would have done it for me.

The Last Performance

I had always imagined it like the premature lowering of a theater curtain on an interesting play …

Slowly, evenly and inexorably reducing our view until nothing was visible but the actors' feet …

Then nothing …

Instead, it is an annoying array of multiple, sheer and sometimes overlapping, tinted scrims …

They are of varying widths, lengths and opacity, hung across the entire proscenium in no discernible pattern …

Each has its own controlling ropes and they lower in random and intermittent order, rate and frequency …

They confuse and distract her and those who observe her, but she continues to perform with grace and bravery …

The audience watches in rapt attention, very proud and, strangely, not really sad …

—Bob Betterton

CONTENTS

Foreword

Former First Lady Nancy Reagan. TV and Broadway star David Hyde Pierce. Princess Yasmin, the daughter of glamorous former film star Rita Hayworth. I have something in common with all of them. So do you. That is why you have this book in your hand.

Each of us has had a loved one ravaged by Alzheimer's Disease. We have helplessly watched them morph from vibrant family members into complete strangers who continue to appear nearly as they had before.

The vast majority of the five million Alzheimer's victims in this country are not celebrities like the three people I mentioned and neither are the families who love them. They are people like you and me, trying to get through this tragedy, while keeping ourselves intact.

Whether you and the victim are just beginning the search for a diagnosis, trying to adjust to its reality, or wondering if what you are doing is the right thing, you are eager for answers. Whether the victim for whom you are caring is in mild early stage, the frustrating for both of you moderate stage or the heartbreaking severe stage you surely have doubts. I have been there and done that.

Caring for an Alzheimer's victim is the Ultimate Do-It-Yourself Project. The problem is that you may think that you are building a sailboat and then it turns out that it has to be a tool shed.

To the astonishment of the Medical Professionals, we were able to keep my wife at home and thriving for thirteen years with moderate to severe Alzheimer's Disease. That was 25% of our married life. To do what we did takes dedication, planning and a large measure of faith. However, we are ordinary people like you and we did it. Many of you can as well.

I wrote this book for one reason. Over those past thirteen years, I have lost track of the number, but this devastating disease touched perhaps close to a hundred friends either as victims or as caregivers. A few weeks ago, I attended my fifty-fifth college reunion and in the space of half an hour heard of three more stricken class-mates. This book is for them, their friends, families, and you.

One of the strange characteristics of Alzheimer's Disease is that each case is different in the sequence and intensity of the debilitation. Because of this, some victims and their caregivers are not good candidates for our approach. However, I am sure that many and perhaps most are as good as we were or better. You will never regret that you at least considered trying it. I have not.

This book is about my wife Mona's struggle with Alzheimer's Disease, but it is not a chronological, day-by-day account of the slow degeneration of the disease. Instead, it is topical and deals with the issues we faced. There are both successes and failures, but happily more of the former.

It is not clear when Mona contracted Alzheimer's, although we now believe it was as much or more than eight years earlier than her formal diagnosis at the age of seventy-one.

Although it is also clear that her memory problems were not always related to Alzheimer's disease perhaps other conditions masked its onset, which means we never really knew where she was in its progression or, more accurately its regression. Regardless of that uncertainty and whatever its cause this has been a journey of her more than thirteen years with dementia.

Since I was convinced that Mona suffered from Alzheimer's long before the initial diagnosis, it did not surprise me when it came. Far more disturbing at that time were the comments from doctors, including psychiatrists and internists that "Unfortunately, she doesn't qualify for a Nursing Home", as if that were bad news. Others said, "You are going to need a great deal of help to get through this", or asked, "Do you have the resources to put her into a care facility so you can have a life of your own?"

None of those comments seemed consistent with the contract to which I agreed more than fifty-two years earlier. In fact, I resented the suggestion that they might be. I felt they were a reflection on my loyalty to my partner in her time of most serious need. Perhaps that reaction was naïve, but I am certain that it would have been hers, had the situation been reversed.

My reaction to these comments related to three principal factors:

- Mona had asked me repeatedly over the years to promise she could live in our home for the rest of her life. I did that and took it literally as a commitment.

- I strongly believed that despite the excellence of the facility into which my mother had moved many years earlier, her quality of life and mental health severely and quickly declined as a direct and adverse result of that move.

- Perhaps selfishly, I also could not imagine that a daily drive to wherever Mona was living would be easier on me than having her near at hand, especially during upstate New York winters.

Therefore, I decided that moving Mona out of the house would be only a last resort. The implementation of that decision, which I still believe was correct, is the subject of this book, written in the hope of encouraging others at least to consider this alternative in an incredibly difficult situation. In that sense, it is a self-help book, although you will not find any formulaic solutions in it.

My approach to Mona's care has been very simple, often to the point of raising serious questions from the medical community and professional caregivers as to it being simplistic, although they have been uniformly amazed at the positive results:

- I believed that Mona's life should remain as close to normal as possible, without making my life any more abnormal than necessary.

- I believed she should have as much freedom as her need for security allows.

- I believed that Mona should be as independent as is acceptably safe.

- I believed I should always be nearby to support and protect, but never be in her face.

Ironically, the Home Health Care Aide who worked with Mona the longest told me she became depressed and guilt ridden when she thought about Mona's condition. Five years earlier, she had moved her father into a care facility and his condition began to deteriorate immediately. She wondered if she had done him a disservice by not doing as we had.

That said, I don't think this course of action is for everyone. It has definitely been the right decision for us. I will leave it to you, the reader to determine whether I have done my job and whether this alternative would work for you. However, there is one more thing for your consideration.

Although the decision to dismiss this approach for all practical purposes becomes irrevocable, to attempt it is not. It may work for a while and then become too onerous. For many, it will work for as long as it did for us. I suspect that for a few, particularly those stronger than I, it will work until the end. The challenge is to make it work for as long as it is the right decision.

—Robert J. Betterton

Acknowledgements

I have some people to thank. First, our children, who keep me grounded and humble, not always in that order: Maryellen and Tom, Paula and Bob, Regi and Jim. Second, our grandchildren and their partners who may sadly also face decisions like this someday: Shannon and Ian, Megan and Dave, Amy and Tommy, Loni and Jamie, Chelsea, Mike, Natalie, Zack and Shelby. Special mention also goes to Mona's Border Collie, Tipper Gorgeous.

I must also acknowledge four other sources of joy, if not yet support, our three great-grandsons, Adrian, Jackson, Connor Robert; our great-granddaughter Ryan Olivia and all those who follow and do not yet realize what, unfortunately, they have missed.

Then there are the medical people: Dr. Betty Rabinowitz, who saved Mona's life at least twice, Drs. Pierre Tariot and Saleem Ismael at the Strong Alzheimer's Unit, and Connie Brand the Nurse conducting the Clinical Trials. There also are my great assistants: the Visiting Nurses and Home Health Care Aides, and Home & Heart Day Care of St. Ann's Community. Then, there is The Friendly Home, which now one might accurately call Mona's Friendly Home.

Finally, there is my best, unrelated friend, Diane Wilmot who has been in charge of my commas, syntax and dangling participles for forty-four years.

CHAPTER 1

▼

DO NOT TAKE "INCONCLUSIVE" FOR A DIAGNOSIS

Around eleven o'clock on a Saturday evening in June 2002 my wife Mona and I left the campus of LeMoyne College in Syracuse, New York and began the ninety-minute drive to our home in Pittsford, a southeastern suburb of Rochester. We had just spent two wonderful, nostalgic days at our fiftieth class reunion.

We met in 1948 as members of the second class graduated from LeMoyne. The college was very small at the time. There were fewer than 250 in our class and even fewer in the only class ahead of us. Everyone knew everyone. Over the years, many of us had kept in close touch and nearly a third of our classmates had been at the reunion.

Reunion Weekend was more memorable because concurrently Mona's sister and her husband were attending their forty-fifth and our daughter Maryellen was up from Atlanta to celebrate her twenty-fifth.

We had greeted many old friends and shared a wealth of experiences. However, heading home before we were three miles down the road Mona asked where we had been. She was pleased when I told her and happy when I answered yes to her question about whether she had seen people she knew. Then she asked if she "had acted all right". I assured her she had.

We rode in silence for a few minutes and then Mona asked softly "Would you tell me all about it?"

For the next hour or so, I went through the whole weekend: the Friday night class party, the picnic on Saturday afternoon and the formal dinner we had just left. I told her what she wore, whom we saw and what we had learned about them.

She listened intently as if she were again a student, attentive to one last review by the professor prior to a semester final exam. Occasionally, she asked a question, sometimes ironically about someone, I hadn't mentioned and who wasn't there, but might have been.

In the darkness, I couldn't tell whether she was sad that she didn't remember, but I sensed that she was pleased that I was helping her. She never asked me about it again.

A few weeks later, a package arrived from the college. It was a group picture of the class members taken at the Friday night party. Mona opened the package and brought me the picture not knowing what it was. We talked about it and she recognized some people, but soon lost interest. She put the picture away and I didn't see it again for more than four years. I found it in a drawer I was cleaning out in anticipation of moving.

When we were at the Reunion, with most of the people she knew I had managed to mention privately and unobtrusively "Mona has a short term memory problem". The response often was "So do I". I did not mention Alzheimer's Disease, even though Mona had been having "a little problem with short term memory" for many years.

In fact, in the early eighties I began to notice that Mona's memory, excellent up to that point was beginning to fail. It was not that this was a serious failure, but it was enough out of character to lead me to make an uninformed judgment that it was the onset of Alzheimer's Disease.

The current wisdom at that time was that one could diagnose Alzheimer's Disease, identified in 1904 by two methods: Elimination of other potential causes or autopsy. Her doctor suggested that we just be conscious of whether it seemed to be getting worse.

Over the next ten years, it slowly became obvious that Mona had a serious drinking problem, culminating in me doing and intervention in December 1993 when she awoke not knowing where she was or what she was doing. During her treatment, the doctors made a diagnosis of Dementia due to Wernicke-Korsakoff syndrome.

Although it is not a definitive medical source Wikopedia, the on-line encyclopedia provides a useful layman's definition and basic information about Dementia and its causes:

> "Dementia is the progressive decline in cognitive function due to damage or disease in the brain beyond what might be expected from normal aging.
> Particularly affected areas may be memory, attention, language and problem solving. Especially in the later stages of the condition, affected persons may be disoriented in time (not knowing what day of the week, day of the month, month, or even what year it is), in place (not knowing where they are), and in person (not knowing who they are).
> Symptoms of dementia can be classified as either reversible or irreversible depending upon the etiology of the disease. Less than 10% of cases of dementia have been reversed. Dementia is a non-specific term encompassing many disease processes, just as fever is attributable to many etiologies.
> Without careful assessment, delirium can easily be confused with dementia and a number of other psychiatric disorders because many of the signs and symptoms are also present in dementia (as well as other mental illnesses including depression and psychosis."

Wikopedia further states that the most common causes of Dementia, in descending order are Alzheimer's Disease, Vascular Infarction (usually heart attack or stroke), Lewy Bodies (also found in Parkinson's Disease), Wernicke-Korsakoff syndrome (also called Alcohol-Induced Persistence Disease) and Frontotemporal Lobar Degeneration (often called Pick's Disease). Less than 5% of a sample of Dementia cases has a potentially treatable cause and with Alzheimer's Disease, that percentage is currently zero.

Wernicke-Korsakoff differs from Alzheimer's and Pick's Diseases because its form of Dementia is not degenerative once the victim stops drinking. In fact, some Wernicke-Korsakoff syndrome victims recover a portion of their lost memory during the first two years of sobriety, although after that period the rest is permanently lost. Therefore, there was no reason to take medication to delay its progression even if it were available, which it wasn't.

At that time, those Dementia cases attributed to Vascular Infarction were only those clinically observed during stroke or heart attacks. Since the cause was traumatic rather than degenerative, once again there seemed to be no reason to take medication.

In 1996, two years after Mona's diagnosis with Dementia due to Wernicke-Korsakoff syndrome I began to see further degeneration in Mona's memory as well as some degradation in Executive Function, which is the ability to perform two or more sequential tasks to produce a desired result. It was not that she could not perform either of the tasks, but that she couldn't seem to see the connection between them. The result was that occasionally she seemed unable to act, which led her to frustration and more confusion.

I had developed an excellent rapport with Mona's Primary Care Physician and I brought these developments to her attention. Over time, she agreed that something different was happening and that we were probably dealing with Alzheimer's, masked by Wernicke-Korsakoff syndrome. As it is today, psychiatrists made diagnoses of Alzheimer's although few of them were deeply involved in Alzheimer's research. I made an appointment for Mona with a well regarded such psychiatrist.

His analysis consisted of reviewing a standard psychological questionnaire, a forty-five minute interview with Mona and a half hour with both of us. He was not interested in my observations and he determined that the evidence of Alzheimer's was inconclusive.

Mona's memory and Executive Function problems continued to worsen and two years later, we repeated the process. The results were the same. Exasperated with the situation and mindful of the serious stress the procedure caused Mona; in 1999, we gave up trying to get an acceptable answer.

What we did not realize and apparently neither did the psychiatrist was that there had been some great advances locally in the identification and diagnosis of Alzheimer's Disease. They were in the use of new technology, specifically MRI and PET brain scans, as well as more sophisticated testing and interview techniques.

More importantly, there were new medications developed through the work of a local psychiatrist and his colleagues across the country. We were clearly barking up the proverbial wrong tree.

This exacerbated the difficulty of diagnosis for Mona, as you will see. For the previous fourteen years she actually had two of the four most common causes of Dementia, Wernicke-Korsakoff syndrome first <u>and later</u> Alzheimer's.

I suspect that this particular phenomenon is common, so it is critically important that one not stop investigating just because of the discovery of one cause. Unfortunately, that was the practice in the early nineties.

At this time, one will not recover from Alzheimer's with or without treatment. However, new medications are under development which when started early, could delay the onset of the most debilitating aspects of the disease and a productive life can be somewhat extended.

Most doctors will not prescribe these medications and most medical plans will not pay for them without the diagnosis by a psychiatrist. As a result, Mona did not receive treatment that might have helped.

Clearly, by the time of our Fiftieth Reunion in June of 2002 Mona's reaction to it indicated that she had much more than "a little problem with short term memory". I think she knew that as well as I. Nevertheless, neither of us knew what to do about it.

A couple months later during my routine annual physical, my doctor saw signs of severe stress in me and asked some probing questions. I told him about Mona and my lack of success in getting a diagnosis, much less treatment for her. He told me about a doctor whom he had met, but did not know well. He said the man had developed a national reputation for his Alzheimer's work.

The man was Pierre N. Tariot, MD. Dr. Tariot was Professor of Psychiatry, of Medicine, of Neurology, and of Aging and Developmental Biology at the University of Rochester Strong Medical Center. He was also the Director of Psychiatry Programs at Monroe Community Hospital in Neurobehavioral Therapeutics. I asked Mona's doctor to arrange an appointment for Mona with Dr. Tariot, and she did, for early December 2002.

Dr. Tariot had reviewed Mona's entire file before he met with her alone for about an hour. Then he had me join them while he did some simple tests. He also asked me a number of questions about what I had observed.

When we were through, Dr. Tariot said he wanted to go over his notes and would be in touch with us. He also requested an MRI brain scan. On December 18, 2002, I received a letter from Dr. Tariot saying that based on his interview with Mona and her test results, including the MRI his diagnosis was that she had Alzheimer's Disease. That was nine years and one week after the intervention for alcoholism and six months after that Reunion weekend.

The experts insist that there is no clinical evidence that Wernicke-Korsakoff's Syndrome can or will develop into Alzheimer's, but I believe that the existence of the Wernicke-Korsakoff diagnosis at least precluded an earlier diagnosis of Alzheimer's. It was just too easy to blame her problems on something, which they could say was not going to get worse.

I felt strangely vindicated and wished, for Mona's sake that we had found Dr. Tariot sooner. I looked forward to the follow up visit scheduled for after the holidays. However, I was also very angry. The earlier psychiatrist should have listened more to the person who knew her best and he did not. I find that to be intellectually arrogant and certainly regrettable, if not professionally inept.

I recognize the problems with trying to make an accurate diagnosis based on some test scores and a brief interview. I also understand the danger of a diagnosis, which results in unwarranted concern and reaction. However, I believe that because of my proximity to the situation and interest in it, I had the diagnosis right perhaps as much as six years earlier than the doctors and maybe more.

I am not sure that for Mona in the end it makes any significant difference, except that she might be much further along in the process of Alzheimer's Disease than one might think. However, as research develops more treatment options, especially in the case of genetic early onset Alzheimer's, that can be critical. There must be more recognition of the intrinsic value of reasonably objective eyewitness testimony and the "system" should allow for that kind of input. Currently, it often does not.

Culpable ignorance is never a good thing. Doctors and other medical professionals have a responsibility at least to consider their non-provable beliefs, and Dr. Tariot did that. If the other doctor had done the same, I would have aggressively searched for a second opinion and we might have found Dr. Tariot earlier.

A number of things can cause temporary memory lapses. The normal aging process makes people more forgetful than they were when they were younger. Moreover, one may later remember things forgotten for the moment, even without trying. One should not jump to conclusions as soon as these behaviors appear.

However, today, there is no excuse for failing to obtain an early diagnosis of Alzheimer's and there are newly discovered clues, which may assist the victim and his or her family to detect early indications.

For example, in a casual conversation with Mona's doctor that I learned that Alzheimer's victims often lose peripheral vision and hearing. That explained why I often startled her by walking into a room, even though I had been around the house and in and out of that room for several hours. Of course, being startled is also the result of the brain failing to process the bits of incomplete information provided by the senses.

Ironically, when we were first married, like her mother, Mona had suffered a severe hearing loss, which a surgical procedure called a stapendectomy corrected. We began to think that the mechanical parts that had been implanted might have failed.

From a different perspective, there is now some research going on into the phenomenon that an inability to identify certain specific odors may be a predictor of Alzheimer's. The list of those that are the best predictors includes strawberry, smoke, soap, menthol, clove, pineapple, natural gas, lilac, lemon and leather. Smoke and natural gas are of course particularly worrisome.

There is also another important reason for seeking a diagnosis as soon as warning signs appear. "Early onset Alzheimer's", affecting the victim before they reach their early to mid-fifties, may actually be a genetic form of the disease, possibly having ramifications for the siblings and children of the victim. Failure to seek a diagnosis could place those siblings in danger, or effectively deny them medication, which could in turn delay the effects of the disease.

Alzheimer's Disease is a terrible thing. However, delaying the seeking of a diagnosis is a disservice to all concerned, especially the victim. One must face Alzheimer's forthrightly because its effect is inevitable and that can be even more traumatic if ignored.

It has been my experience from the day my wife was diagnosed with Alzheimer's, that when I told one of our female friends about it; I would occasionally receive the response "My husband has it too". However, when I asked if he had been diagnosed the answer was, more often than not, that he hadn't. Since there is no cure what difference did it make, they would say.

Ironically, I have never had any male friend say to me, "My wife has it too, but she has not been diagnosed". The fact is that 70% of the diagnosed Alzheimer's victims are women.

Perhaps the explanation for this discrepancy is because the diagnosis of Alzheimer's Disease is one of the most feared, not just because of the terrifying aspects of the disease itself, but also because of vanity regarding the connotation that the victim is getting old and perhaps more women than men fear that. We are a youth oriented culture and as a result, the fearful victims devise elaborate strategies to mask their memory loss in a vain effort to hide their aging process, as if they could.

Although I cannot speak from personal experience, it is logical to assume that the first person to become aware of approaching Dementia is the victim. Who can forget the terror portrayed by Henry Fonda in the movie "On Golden Pond" when his character became disoriented and lost in a familiar forest surrounding his long time summer home?

Denial is perhaps a rational response for the victim. However, that does not excuse enabling by friends and family.

I can tell you from experience that Alzheimer's victims can become accomplished actors, working very hard to cover mistakes and rarely admitting to things that others did not witness. Their friends, and particularly their families, often become compassionate, unwitting enablers.

Friends and family members sometimes give the victim wide latitude out of misplaced love or affection, perhaps because of the fear that they will have to become caregivers or worse yet, may also become victims. This conspiracy by the victim, family, friends and sometimes the doctor, combined with imprecise diagnostic tools, often results in a late diagnosis.

Personally, I suspect that other failures to diagnose in a timely manner may really be the result of factors other than medical. Certainly, the insurance industry is not anxious to identify more people needing care and doctors are not looking for more families to blame them when their patients don't get better. If you don't diagnose it, you don't have to treat it, so when you don't know how to reverse it, why identify it?

It is also true that most families intuitively want to delay institutionalization for as long as possible. What they fail to realize is that institutionalization is often not an immediate reality and in fact, may not even be an available option.

Until there is a cure, or at least an assurance that the regression of the disease can be arrested or somewhat reversed, most of these attitudes will not change. However, that does nothing to allay the frustration of loved ones and victims who know something is wrong and only suspect what it is.

CHAPTER 2

▼

GETTING ON WITH IT

The diagnosis of Mona's Alzheimer's Disease was actually anti-climactic. It was essentially an affirmation of what we already knew and had at least partially accepted. However, it also was a perverse opportunity for me to angrily shout the "I told you so" that I never wanted to utter. Strangely, I didn't feel up to that and did not.

It is not only proper to grieve when one learns that a loved one is afflicted with Dementia but, in fact, it would be unnatural if one did not. The person you knew so well is no longer the person who looks like him or her, sitting across the table. The person you knew has gone in a way similar to death, despite the Theological problems inherent in the analogy.

My grief hit me in a store in 1993 when Mona was in the hospital undergoing rehab, but already obviously afflicted with Wernicke-Korsakoff Syndrome. It continued in the car as I drove home through tears and ran its course over many sleepless nights, alone.

I am sure that Mona grieved as well, but internalized it more. I also assume her grief was somewhat less selfish, concerned more with the impact on others. However, one of the few, albeit ironic benefits of Alzheimer's Disease is that eventually the victim forgets even grief.

I am not sure that anyone who has not been through this process can really ever understand it. We are all too accustomed to the belief that "if there is life, there is still hope". Unfortunately, for victims of Alzheimer's and many other diseases there is no hope for a cure, only for the strength to endure the inevitable. The profile of that reality varies from disease to disease, and I make no judgment about the relative devastation brought about by any of them in particular.

I have been to the funerals of at least two women and two men who died of Alzheimer's. All were in good marriages, but their spouses were not grieving in the usual sense. Some people remarked that one of the husbands seemed relieved rather than sad, and that "the reality of her death will probably hit him hard later".

I don't agree. I am sure that the reality had hit him much earlier, probably years before. For him now it was far more like attending a memorial service than a funeral. I also suspect that like me, when he had grieved, there was no one around to comfort him.

Others had to grieve as well. Although our children were close enough to the situation to have done pretty much as I had, some extended family members still had not fully accepted that Mona was as severely impaired as she really was. It was a while before they did.

The best time to do one's grieving is when the effects of Alzheimer's are first manifested, for two solid reasons. First, it is affirmation that the process has started, is irreversible and one's acceptance of that reality has begun. Second, getting through the grief frees one to deal in an unimpaired way with the problems to be faced immediately, for the rest of your common life and years after that, far more objectively and practically.

Ecclesiastes had it right. There is a time to grieve. Nevertheless, there is also a time to get off your duff, stand on your own two feet and get on with things. I guess, in a way, that is what some people try to express with that strange word, closure.

Unlike with death, getting on with things involves often being in the presence of someone who looks almost exactly like the person for whom you have already grieved. That kind of closure takes some doing.

The primary purpose of this book is to assist others in dealing with that process in a pro-active rather than a passive fashion. People ask me if I have written a "self-help" book and I have always said that wasn't possible. There is no traditional "self-help" book for Alzheimer's. This book is about how Mona and I approached her disease. If it helps some to develop their own approaches, I am very pleased.

Mona's diagnosis did provide an occasion for reflection on where we might be in this journey, what we knew about the disease and ourselves, what we had to do, and ultimately, where all of that would take us. The unrelated and incomplete assumptions we had made became tangible realities and we both had to deal with them.

It was, at the same time, too early and too late for an orderly discussion of the future. We hadn't yet contemplated the enormity of the situation and we didn't really know enough about the details of the disease to form any real opinions. This situation was further complicated by the fact that it seemed like all anyone wanted to talk about, at least to me, was institutionalizing.

I suppose that it is natural for them to do that, but I was surprised that one of the first things the medical professionals brought up after making the diagnosis was eligibility for and availability of institutionalized care. A major decision point was now upon us and at least I knew that once made, it was irrevocable.

There are many living arrangement options available for people facing the decisions we were, especially if cost is not a consideration. However, neither of us had ever expressed any particular interest in exploring any of them, except if one or the other of us ultimately reached the point of absolute necessity.

I realize that many of my readers are aware of what I am about to explain. However, if you are not, you need to be. I will try to be as clear and concise as I can.

There is a broad spectrum of residence options available to the elderly these days, ranging from "retirement villages" to "nursing homes". They represent many levels of service and care.

The intervening levels of care often have euphemistic names like "independent living", "assisted living", "enhanced care", and "enriched care" and each has a different cost associated with the confusing name. Certain levels of care, including "assisted living", must be licensed and meet specified standards. Those standards, however, are often related merely to minimums of safety, security and hygiene.

We have all read about abuses of residents by unqualified, untrained and sometimes unscrupulous staff. Some of these are criminal and all are tragic.

Although people often use the term incorrectly, Nursing Homes (officially Skilled Nursing Facilities) are the most clearly defined facilities, in that they must have on-site medical facilities and a minimum number of Registered Nurses available 24 hours a day. They also have stringent qualification requirements. Medicare and Medicaid only cover this care level.

The confusion arises because many Nursing Homes separate patients with Dementia problems like Alzheimer's Disease from the rest of their population, and Assisted Living facilities do the same thing. They do this in both venues principally because the danger of Alzheimer's victims wandering is greater than that of the other patients.

Some "assisted living" facilities have what they call "Alzheimer's Units", "Dementia Units" or "Memory Units". These units are not required to have medical facilities or 24-hour professional presence. They are merely areas of the facility distinguished by sophisticated lockdown capabilities to prevent the Alzheimer's victims from wandering.

At the time of her diagnosis, Mona was found to be in the Moderate Stage of Alzheimer's, unqualified for Nursing Home care and therefore ineligible for Medicare or Medicaid coverage. As I write this, although Mona is in the Advanced Severe stage, she is still not clearly qualified for anything more than assisted living. That is determined, at least in New York State by a PRI evaluation, administered by a trained and approved Registered Nurse.

While I had lived in many houses for the first twenty-three years of my life, Mona had lived in only one and her grandfather had built it. We lived in an apartment during the three years while I was on active duty in the Navy and then we moved in with Mona's parents for a year. We spent just six years in our first house, and as I write this, we have lived in our current home for forty-two years, well over half of each of our lives.

In those forty-two years, hardly a day has passed, including since her diagnosis, when Mona hasn't said how much she loves our home and wants to stay in it forever. Forever is not in the cards, but I knew what our first decision had to be.

I had determined that the criterion for Mona entering institutional care would be very simple: When, and only then, I could no longer provide her with the care she required at home.

There were a number of factors, which went into that decision:

- In effect, Mona had asked me to do that.
- I believed her care was my job and that I could do it.
- Mona did not require skilled nursing care.
- I was keenly aware of the negative effect of moving my mother from her home.
- Selfishly, the distance I would have to travel to see her could be onerous.

Another factor in the decision process trumped everything else: What I would do for her had to be no less than what she would have done for me. Such a choice is definitely not for everyone, and I would not make a judgment about anyone else's decision to the contrary.

As I think you will see, the decision was right for us. The medical professionals are amazed at the way Mona has been able to maintain her functionality, sociability and happiness level despite her decline into the advanced stages of this terrible disease. It is their opinion that this would not have been possible if she had gone into any kind of care facility at the outset.

This book is about how Mona and I together at first, with the help of many others have made this decision work. We are not unique. Under the right conditions, many people should be able to do the same thing. However, they must make that decision for themselves.

Major changes have been required. Obviously, some have been physical. Others, though sometimes appearing complex, have been merely operational. However, perhaps the most important changes have been philosophical. I will describe the three classes of changes in this chapter and develop them more fully in the rest of the book.

Remember however, this is not a how-to-do-it manual. It is just what has worked and in some cases not worked for us.

Physical Environment Changes

The safety and security of the victim may dictate the need for physical changes to implement such a decision. Fortunately for us, these changes were minimal, mostly because Mona did not exhibit any propensity to wander and she was not confrontational, two common traits of Alzheimer's victims. The presence of either of those traits would have put our decision into serious question.

Our home is located in a quiet, suburban development in the Town of Pittsford, New York on a street that does not exit the tract. To leave the tract requires traveling on a minimum of two other streets and the route is not intuitive. It is unlikely that Mona could get out of the tract in less than fifteen minutes and she is not inclined to try. Of course, that could change, but initially I decided that no special measures or changes to prevent her wandering were necessary.

Our neighbor on one side moved in at the same time we did forty-two years ago. On the other side is a relative newcomer of about thirty-five years. I made sure that they were aware of the situation.

With the exception of outdoor grilling, we do all our cooking with electricity. Therefore, neither escaping gas nor explosions are of concern, although there certainly is the possibility of a range surface fire. Of less concern is the slightly more remote possibility of a toaster fire. Vigilance is the answer here, but Mona has become less and less inclined over recent years to attempt any cooking at all.

From the outset, I considered it within the proper level of safety and security to allow Mona free access to all areas on the main and second floors, the garage and the backyard. She is discouraged from going into the basement, simply by eliminating any reasons to do so and rarely, if ever, does. That assessment is the same today. Nonetheless, I monitor all of this very closely.

Operational Changes

I made these changes for efficiency and control, and most of those necessary are in this area. Some like taking over the driving, financial management and shopping chores were part of our life before Mona's diagnosis, and for about a year, I had been doing most of the cooking.

I had also taken over the details of her scheduling, particularly her medications and health care. More and more it has extended to managing her wardrobe, supervising her dressing and doing the laundry.

These changes will continue as Mona's capabilities diminish, but I think it is important for many reasons that "taking over" just because it is easier than not, should be resisted as long as possible. This maintains the victim's dignity as well as independence.

I have tried to develop an attitude in dealing with Mona of treating her as if she were slightly less impaired than she really is, and at the same time being ready to provide assistance if she needs it. I try to help her gently to refuse to give up without trying.

Philosophical Changes

The need for philosophical changes is far subtler than the others are and the Carekeeper is affected significantly more than the victim is. The Carekeeper must learn to embrace things counter-intuitive. For example, he or she needs to re-evaluate the efficacy of self-sacrifice. He or she must learn to ignore some things and concentrate on others. They must change without losing touch with themselves. If this doesn't happen, the project will fail and there will have been two victims of this disease.

This is not to say that the victim does not purposefully change and fight to maintain control, especially in the earlier stages when they are striving desperately to hang on to their essence. Some of the things they do are very creative.

Initially, Mona placed increased importance on surrounding herself with pictures of family. However, those pictures were taken at many different times and we are a group with strong family resemblances. Subsequently, those helpful and comforting photos began to contribute to her confusion with generations, identities and relationships all becoming unrecognizable.

Of all the things related to the onset of her Dementia, I was the least prepared for the speed and intensity with which Mona became dependent on me. Although after she came back from rehab at Conifer Park in 1994 she was quite dependent, after a while that seemed to lessen. Nevertheless, by 2002, I had become her memory, her decision maker and the interpreter of the world around her.

For reasons unrelated to Mona's condition, nearly two and a half years before her diagnosis, I had made significant changes in my business, scaling back its scope and relocating my office to our daughter's former bedroom on the second floor of our home. In a way this was very fortuitous, because it provided me a closer view of Mona's deteriorating condition.

I continued to work full time in my business of producing professional corporate golf outings at five star resorts across the country wherein the corporations, with which I worked could entertain their most important clients and customers. However, use of these events is highly susceptible to changing business conditions and economic slow downs severely affected us.

Then came September 11, 2001, and large-scale business entertaining, especially that involving air travel, virtually came to a halt. In my business, since the people with whom I dealt were themselves often victims of the situation and had lost their jobs, recovery usually meant starting from scratch, with new people, new relationships and new decision makers.

To facilitate re-establishment of relationships would have required me to travel extensively and that would have been a problem. Mona's diagnosis made it was clear that unless she entered a care facility my principal occupation was her care.

This shift in emphasis established a degree of freedom in adapting to my responsibilities related to Mona's condition. However, I did continue to spend the majority of my time in my office. It became a haven, to which I could retreat to regroup and try to preserve my own mental health.

I returned to my high school dream of writing and this new activity kept me from being always in Mona's face, allowing her to maintain some level of her formerly extensive independence and privacy. I jealously guarded "my space" and made it clear to Mona that when she was there it was as a guest. For the most part, at least for a time, she understood and respected that.

Without a doubt, the most devastating result of Dementia is the loss of intimacy. I don't mean physical intimacy, although considerable guilt about that aspect of one's life quickly emerges. I mean the intimacy of shared references, of not having to explain a humorous remark; of knowing what a partner's reaction will be before it occurs, of easily understanding the complex meaning of a look or simple gesture. Those are only the minor and earliest losses.

I believed that Mona was not ready to talk about how she felt. I knew that I didn't know enough about where we stood, what the future held and what I could or couldn't do, to give her any real guidance. Throughout the prior nine years, we made many accommodations in our lives because of Mona's Dementia related memory problems.

We made these changes evolutionally, without the benefit of a diagnosis any more specific than "inconclusive", and we were comfortable with those decisions. However, we were beginning to realize a good deal of what we had done was an exercise in naïveté.

For five or more years, I had been functioning as Mona's memory and had gradually become responsible for making many of her decisions, large and small, not because I chose to, but because she asked and I knew I had to do it. Therefore, it wasn't a dramatic event when we had "an official diagnosis". In effect, I had already become both of us, which is quite different from both of us becoming one.

The great irony is that this dependence begins as a team effort, with victim and his or her partner working together. I can hear you saying, "Okay, what is the big deal about that"? The "big deal" is that, in most team situations, team members learn more and more about how to work together. As a result, they become increasingly able to pick up the slack for one another and the team performance actually becomes better than merely the sum of their individual efforts. That is not the case in this disease.

The victim becomes less and less able to contribute to the effort. In fact, at least in Mona's case, the victim may begin to adopt behavior that is counter-productive, actually making the task more difficult, which accelerates the breakdown of the process to the point where one teammate has essentially ceased to contribute to completing the task. Soon the victim actually seems to be an opponent, rather than a teammate. That diminishes team's net performance. Half of two has become much less than one.

For example, one day I walked into the kitchen to replenish my morning coffee and found Mona in tears, trying to fill her daily-compartmented, weekly pillbox. I showed her how to line up all her pills for Sunday and then repeat that six more times before putting any in the box.

That worked fine until one day I realized that Mona had started refilling the day's compartment as soon as she took the pills that were in it and, therefore, she could not tell whether she had taken them or not. That defeated the primary purpose of the box.

I think I have a reasonable level of facility with the English language. However, although I tried mightily, I could not explain that concept to her. Mona knew she must refill the compartments. One was empty, so she filled it. I had to take possession of the prescription bottles and the pillbox, and begin to control completely the distribution of her medications.

If I had not been working at home, I might not have been aware of this problem for months, but because I was on-site, I could deal with the problem as it developed. However, there is a danger in this. The tendency becomes to just take over a task when, for at least a little while longer, a little coaching is all that is really required. In such cases, taking over is an unnecessary burden, albeit minor at the outset for the Carekeeper, but it can be devastating to the victim's self-esteem.

In addition, sometimes the change in responsibility is traumatic because of the difference in approach to implementation between the victim and the Carekeeper. An excellent example of this comes readily to mind.

Without being sexist about it, I am confident that my background and business experience has made me more organized, disciplined and efficient in approaching many tasks than even Mona was, although I had always been careful never to impose my way on her. Therefore, I suspect that I do some elements of Mona's share with less effort than she needed. I also feel that because of necessity in my business life, I learned as much about multi-tasking and time management as Mona had to develop in operating our home and raising three children. I think that for us, this is merely a cultural difference rather than one of either gender or intellect.

We often joked about there being men's work and women's work, although those distinctions were really based on which things each preferred (or disliked the least) to contribute in the larger context of accomplishing the common work to be done. However, we never second-guessed each other about the way in which we did the work we accepted.

I remember an incident that occurred in the first year of our marriage and illustrates this point well. We were living in a tiny, one bedroom apartment in Washington, DC. It was a "Pullman apartment" because the rooms were arranged one behind one another like cars on a train, connected by a hallway, which ran directly from the front door to the kitchen in the rear and through that opened onto a very small back porch.

We had a little party one evening with three other couples, to announce that Mona was pregnant, and it ran rather late. When the guests left, the place was a mess, but I insisted that we were going to bed and that in the morning, since it was Saturday, I would clean the place thoroughly, all by myself.

True to my word, early the next day I began the clean up. Fortunately, I started before Mona was up because my first act was to throw all the empty cans and bottles on the living room floor and to follow that by dumping the contents of all the ashtrays in the same place.

Armed with a stiff bristled push broom, I started at the front door and began to push all the refuse toward the back porch. As I passed the bathroom, our bedroom and the kitchen, I added to the pile, eventually dumping it all in the trashcan on the back porch.

Then I returned to the living room with a tray, for another pass through the apartment. This time I collected dishes and glasses, and deposited the filled tray on the counter next to the sink. On my third trip, I vacuumed while dusting as I went, with a cloth I carried in my left hand. Once that was finished, I washed and put away the dishes and glasses. Three trips through and the apartment was clean. Mona would have approached the job quite differently and perhaps better.

Nearly fifty years later, I was now applying my same approaches to many things Mona had done her way, hopefully with as little trauma as possible. However, I decided I would leave all tasks related to housekeeping in Mona's hands as long as possible.

That decision carried with it the responsibility to accept that it would take her longer than it did previously, that it sometimes wouldn't be done well and that some integral parts would not be done at all. Coaching compensated somewhat, but often I had to complete the task. However, I always tried to do that when she wasn't present.

There was not much discussion between us about the division of responsibility, although in fact, we had already made some other significant changes. As I have said, two of those were shopping and cash management, which had in effect, been made when Mona entered the hospital in 1993.

Ironically, if I had paid more attention to the latter in the years prior to that I might have recognized her difficulties earlier. As it was, straightening out some of the results of Mona's management of our financial resources took a great deal of painful effort over several years.

Shopping was another matter. I have never understood either recreational shopping or impulse buying, so I summarily eliminated both, saving a great deal of time and energy, as well as cash.

The difference between us on this subject was very simple and basic. Mona shopped to find things she might want to buy, whether she needed them or not. I shop only for things, which I <u>must</u> buy because I <u>already</u> need them, often desperately, which I feel is the only true test of need.

At first, Mona still felt comfortable attacking a Mall by herself, so sometimes, after clearly establishing when and where we would meet; I would drop her off for an hour or two. Over time however, it became clear that she was becoming uncomfortable in doing that and by the time she was diagnosed with Alzheimer's we had stopped it.

In a sense, that amounted to the closing of an important chapter in Mona's life. It was not about shopping, but about independence and the confidence in one's ability to take care of one's self.

On the other hand, I had been doing most of the grocery shopping for several years and was very comfortable with that, since for six years while in high school and college, I had worked in a grocery store. I understood the philosophy of store design and there are large areas of the place that I never enter while Mona always wanted to see everything. When we shopped with me in charge, Mona was just along for the ride.

Soon, however, Mona became very detached from the process as the obsessive, compulsive side of her disease began to take over. She began to spend her time straightening store shelves. That led to her falling behind and she would suddenly realize that she didn't know where I was.

When our children were very young, we drilled into them that when they felt they were lost, they should immediately go to the front of the store and wait for us between the checkout counters and the front door. Mona remembered that and I didn't have to worry about her wandering off at least as long as she could sense when she was lost.

I suspect that the randomness of the progress of the disease makes its victims like fingerprints and snowflakes. There are no two alike. Each day brings new challenges, although one begins to see patterns and relationships as new symptoms appear and develop.

My cousin sent me a book called "A Promise Kept" by a former President of Columbia Bible College, Robertson McQuilken, in which he tells of his experiences with his wife, following her diagnosis with Alzheimer's Disease. Obviously, the reason my cousin sent me the book was that she assumed my life had, or would become, much the same.

The fact of the matter is that, at least up to that point, I was not able to identify very much with the things he faced. During the period covered by the book, his wife seemed to have a less severe loss of memory and function, although she was constantly wandering off, often for significant periods of time and in situations that threatened her safety. She definitely had a propensity to wander that was far greater than Mona's was. However, with all due respect, he was clueless about how to deal with that and he didn't seem to learn much as he went along.

This is not rocket science. It is the application of patient wisdom to protect the victim's safety and maintain his or her quality of life.

As I write this book, Mona has just begun to present the challenge of wandering, although that is the most commonly reported behavior of Alzheimer's victims. Mona is almost the opposite, always concerned that she will lose her support system, me, even in familiar surroundings.

When she must be on her own, for example to visit a public ladies room, her first action when coming out is to stop and look around for me. I always position myself where I can easily be seen and watch the door. When she emerges, I extend my arm as high as possible over my head and she responds. This reaction may change over time, but for now the system works. However, remember that there is no definitive survival manual for Alzheimer's victims or their Carekeepers.

The biggest changes we made before her diagnosis were in managing Mona's health care, with me sitting in on all testing and examinations, ordering and dispensing of medications, and scheduling her appointments outside the home. I also took over the task of keeping track of family birthdays and anniversaries, although some would say I do a very poor job with that. Once those things began to happen, Mona became more and more dependent on me.

It is my belief that it is good for the victim of Dementia to be urged to do things, even when they have to be helped. However, sometimes that means that I must do the tasks over and at times an immediate intervention is in the interest of health and safety.

Therefore, I unobtrusively began to monitor and to help with the cooking, whenever that was required, but she continued to do the clean up, the laundry and, strangely, taking out the trash, even though that presented an opportunity for her to wander. She was eager to do these things, because they made her feel that she was contributing.

I also made a conscious decision to keep Mona visible, and as far as possible, involved. I rarely attend social activities or events without her, and I urge her to interact with friends we randomly meet. I do this without embarrassment because I am confident that it is the best thing for Mona's continued functionality. She seems to enjoy and appreciate the opportunity for social contact.

To facilitate the interaction, I always try to make those situations as comfortable as I can for all who are involved. To do that I remind Mona of the name of the person she is approaching and how she knows them. I also, as discreetly as possible, try to make the other person aware of Mona's condition. They always seem grateful for that.

Socialization is important and that victims should remain in familiar surroundings with access to family and friends as long as possible. However, it is self-destructive if one prolongs that period to the detriment of the physical or mental health of the victim's family. Implicit in that is a complex decision making process.

For Mona, the future consisted of doing the best she can, for as long as she is able. In a later chapter, I will discuss the ways Mona has done that and her dogged determination to participate fully in her own life, through sheer will. However, Mona has become limited to living completely in the present, in fact in the very moment, without her past for reference and no resources to predict or control her future.

There were more adjustments and accommodations to make and I made them. I decided to make them as subtly as I could, preferably without Mona realizing the effect.

My instincts had told me that allowing her to drive was not a good idea and I took care of that when she first suffered Dementia from the effects of Wernicke-Korsakoff Syndrome. Moreover, my task was to ensure that her physical health remained good, to provide her a safe living environment, and to assist her through this ordeal, while maintaining her quality of life … and mine.

I also feel it is important to maintain Mona's self-esteem and confidence by gently urging her to do all that she could possibly do for herself. Sometimes I have to let her fail, albeit on my terms.

Therefore, as strange as it may seem, the day after a diagnosis of Alzheimer's Disease was very much like the day before. There was no hastily planned trip to the hospital for treatment. No new tests were scheduled. There was no need to awaken at six in the morning to have temperatures and blood pressures taken. Nor was there any other bothersome monitoring by medical professionals. There were no IVs, no therapy and no sense of urgency. There was not even a handi-capped-parking sticker. And no hope.

Mona and I accepted the diagnosis quietly, she for her own unknown reasons, and I, because I had fully anticipated it. Mona had never used the word Alzheimer's with regard to herself and has not to this day. I don't think that is strictly denial because she has readily admitted and accepted her inability to remember and to do certain things.

Perhaps out of defiance or pride, which she had exhibited long before the diagnosis, Mona knew what was happening to her, but would not formally name it because that was giving in. Therefore, the diagnosis was less traumatic for her than one might expect. On reflection, maybe that is denial.

We also didn't really talk about the diagnosis, but we both fully understood. Forty-eight years of marriage will do that. I am certain that Mona understood that her memory problems were going to increase until she became completely helpless. She knew that she would have to rely on me more and more. Mona also trusted, without question, that I would provide that assistance.

An ironic benefit for the victim of Alzheimer's Disease is that unlike other illnesses, once afflicted, their care ceases to be their problem. There is little or no medicine to take or not take. They have no diet to observe or not observe. There are no exercises to do or skip. It is just not their problem.

At first, this is frustrating for the victim. However, experts point out that over time it is the nature of the disease that the victims become happier. Unfortunately, for the Carekeeper that is not the case.

Care and treatment of the victim are the problem of the healthy spouse of a person with Alzheimer's. That's just the way it works. Remember the contract about "in sickness and in health" and "for better or for worse". You made that deal. This is the "sickness and worse" time. Some people, like your children, other relatives and friends, may try to help, but you have to suck it up and face your problem. Have no doubts, it can be handled, but I won't tell you it is easy.

It always struck me as strange that the words caretaker and caregiver mean the same thing, like flammable and inflammable, but in this new role in my relationship with Mona, I realized that neither word accurately described my primary responsibility. Both have the connotation of a series of discrete actions, with intervening periods of non-involvement. My responsibility and that of my many counterparts was far more than that.

When it comes to Alzheimer's victims, as with infants, and I am sure, a number of other situations, the defining responsibility is one of ***Carekeeping***. Carekeeping is a constant awareness, just like lighthouse keeping. An infant progresses and eventually requires less Carekeeping, so caregiving and caretaking become more apt descriptions. An Alzheimer's victim may begin with caregivers and care-takers, but he or she soon regresses and Carekeeping is increasingly essential.

It is also true that although caregiving and caretaking duties can be shared or delegated, Carekeeping cannot. If one is a Carekeeper, one can and usually does, act as a caregiver or caretaker, at least from time to time, but ultimately there can only be one Carekeeper. That Carekeeper cannot wonder what the victim is doing at any point in time, he or she must know. This is not a part-time job. This is a complete immersion in a new, demanding way of life. It can be rewarding, however and even ennobling.

Make no mistake; a diagnosis of Alzheimer's Disease is a fatal conclusion. Although it may not introduce any major changes in medication or treatment, it is a life changing moment. The insidious regression of the disease is gradual and uneven. It moves in many directions, affecting all aspects of the lives of the patient and the family, which may not be readily apparent. If one is not vigilant before long, the disease takes charge and everyone goes into a reactive mode. Avoid that situation at all costs.

The defenses against that condition are a determination to manage the situa-tion, an effort to obtain as much information as can be gathered and the develop-ment of a sophisticated plan to deal with the victim's struggle with the disease. That three-pronged effort must begin immediately. Establish priorities although those may not be as obvious as one might think.

With regard to the first defense, from the outset I have been fiercely commit-ted to the management of Mona's struggle with Alzheimer's Disease for as long as I can do that effectively. I have been equally determined to do that in our home, because I believe that kind of an environment is most beneficial for the victim as long as he or she can function independently.

Having made that statement, I feel I should say that I am also determined to not persist in this task when to do so would not be in Mona's best interest. This book covers that period, which is as long as I, as the Carekeeper, am able to keep the care safely and effectively.

Part of that task includes developing the criteria for the decision to make a change in the care Mona needs when that is appropriate, another element for which there is very little guidance and perhaps no right or wrong course of action. There should be no guilt attached to doing the best one can and then deciding one cannot do more. Never allow this terrible disease to claim more than one vic-tim when it strikes. I will say much more about this subject in a later chapter.

In the ensuing chapters, I will discuss how the division of responsibilities between us has evolved since diagnosis, for all aspects of Mona's life. However, this is not a guidebook. Her needs and capabilities have determined the changes we found necessary, but each Alzheimer's victim is different.

It would be logical for the reader to ask at this point whether assistance is available in identifying the necessary changes to be made in one's life and what to do about that. I asked myself that question and was surprised at what I found.

I will readily admit that at the time they made Mona's diagnosis, my knowledge of Alzheimer's Disease was meager and I needed to correct that as soon as possible. I first turned to the most logical place, the Alzheimer's Association.

The Alzheimer's Association provides a large number of very valuable services and, as far as I know, does them very well. However, one must realize that its principal mission, as with all such organizations, is to raise funds to support medical research into the Disease and to provide awareness and advocacy in the form of lobbying on a number of issues. Within that context, they conduct extensive outreach programs for victims, their families and caregivers in the form of seminars, training sessions and information in a variety of media. I have no quarrel with that hierarchy of values.

My interest was in three specific areas: what I needed to know about keeping Mona safe and healthy, how her needs were going to change, and on what kind of a general timetable. I found that at least at that time there was very little specific information available, not because the organization was not trying, but because that is the nature of the Disease.

I thoroughly read all the material they sent me. I explored the Internet extensively. I asked a large number of questions of her doctor, the psychiatrist and anyone else who I thought might have some insights. I also signed up for some seminars.

I found that the seminars were of three types: general information for victims, family members and caregivers in the early stages; support groups for each of those classifications; and training programs for professional caregivers involved in the care of victims in the more advanced stages of the disease.

I suspect that my reaction to these offerings may not be typical, but on the chance that it is, I will describe it. I found the general information seminar to be useful, but one session was clearly enough. The real information was self-explanatory, but the group participation was less rewarding since it consisted of anecdotal information and since, as I later learned individual cases of Alzheimer's are often very different, I could not identify with most of it.

I admit to a bias in that I am significantly less convinced of the value of support groups when it comes to things other than cases of addictive behavior modification. I am certainly not a psychologist, but with alcohol, drugs, or even anger and gambling, there is a sense of providing inspiration to prevail over one's addiction, which is uplifting. I think such groups for those afflicted in those ways are very helpful, if not essential. Perhaps that is also true for mild to moderate Alzheimer's victims. I just don't know.

Informational meetings for the families, friends, associates and caregivers of these people may be helpful. However, there is just so much one can learn. Therefore, to consider these groups as regular and endless commitments becomes yet another exercise in wallowing in one another's misery and non-productivity, perhaps leading to depression. I feel it is more beneficial for all concerned just to get on with the job.

My reaction to caregiver training to deal with severe Alzheimer's Disease is mixed. It is certainly useful for the professional caregiver and some unique non-professionals, especially if they possess related skills like nursing. I didn't feel that I needed it yet. I also am not convinced that care of Alzheimer's victims in the Severe Stage is appropriate for non-professionals.

I really believe and often say that Alzheimer's Disease is the Ultimate Do-It-Yourself-Project. If you can do it, you will. If you need extensive training, perhaps someone else should be doing it.

Subsequent to the acceptance of the diagnosis of Alzheimer's Disease and one's emergence as the Carekeeper, the first task is to make an objective assessment the needs and to begin formalizing a plan and a support team. In this regard, it is important to remember that the Carekeeper can never assign portions of the basic responsibility, only the execution of the implementing tasks. It is also important in the earlier stages to request no more help than you really need. You may need much more of that help later.

The secret, as with many things, is sophisticated and detailed planning, which is far more than the creation of a To Do List. In addition, remember that planning is a process and one that does not end. The plan is never complete and must be constantly monitored and refined.

The key for the Carekeeper is anticipation and prevention, which means literally assuming constant responsibility for every possible aspect of the health, safety and life of the Alzheimer's victim. That reminds me, you may have noticed that I have not used the term "Alzheimer's patient" and will not knowingly do so in the future. In my mind, a patient is one undergoing recuperative treatment with the expectation of a cure. A victim is simply not that.

Disabuse yourself of the concept of a cure. That is probably not going to happen in our lifetimes and, believe it or not, accepting that reality makes it easier to do what you have to do, because you are not always looking for signs of improvement that are not going to appear.

The best medicine for a Carekeeper is a strong dose of reality. I was pretty naïve about the general subject of Dementia and Alzheimer's in particular, but that is to me, to be expected. There is no way for you to really learn about it until you have lived with it on a 24/7/365 basis.

I clearly understood and accepted the simple definition of my responsibility. I was going to have to learn in a limited sense at first, to manage, if not live, two lives. In time, eventually I would have to do that completely. If I were going to do that task successfully, I needed to organize both of us and I had to do that quickly.

I will admit that although I have been a planner all my life, the importance of this task was now a bit daunting. I wondered if I had the resources to do the job. I began to have serious self-doubt about whether my approach to the problem was correct; whether I knew enough about the task I was facing, and whether I could really accomplish what was necessary. In a word, I was frightened. Scared to death may be closer to the truth.

Because it is a part of who and what I am, I turned to my faith. My personal version of that faith is that there really isn't much need for petitionary prayer, and especially in this case such an exercise is generally ineffective anyway. Short of a miracle, Alzheimer's Disease is not curable and the odds against eliciting a miracle are not worth spending much time considering it unless you have nothing better to do. I did.

One day I ran into an old friend in a store and he asked how Mona was. His face grew more somber as I told him, and then suddenly, he put his hand on my shoulder and solemnly spoke a personalized version of that inane platitude I heard from the Nuns, growing up, "Don't worry, God never gives us a greater burden than we can carry. Just pray".

I politely informed him that he could be find remnants of that theory easily in the pastures, which surround nearly every dairy farm barn in the world. I don't think that is even good Theology to say nothing about not being very reassuring. Actually, I believe that the reverse is true.

I believe that God provides us all with generous amounts of most, if not all of the things we need to get through this life and He constantly replenishes the supply as we use it, especially if we did not squander it. Therefore, rather than bothering God with redundant requests I should decide what I needed and try to figure out where He put it.

My needs came down to patience and wisdom. I understood about patience. The big dictionary on my desk defines wisdom as "intelligence, drawing on experience, governed by prudence". That seemed simple enough and I decided to assume that during the prior seventy-two years, God had provided enough intelligence, experience and prudence for me to mix up a sizable batch of wisdom. Now I just pray I will use my wisdom wisely, as patiently as possible, and very well.

I was now ready to develop the plan. In the ensuing chapters, I will discuss the specifics of my planning to achieve these objectives. Just remember that one plan does not fit all.

CHAPTER 3

▼

DON YOUR OWN OXYGEN MASK BEFORE ASSISTING OTHERS

In order to develop any viable plan, one must first define objectives and establish specific and achievable interim goals. In the case of Mona's struggle with Alzheimer's Disease, those objectives seemed very simple:

- Manage Mona's physical health and safety in a comfortable, familiar environment.

- Do that in a way, which preserves an acceptable quality of her life for as long as possible.

- Establish the criteria for deciding when others could better handle her care.

The interim goals of the plan seemed to be equally simple, although perhaps not as obvious.

The first goal is that I safeguard and maintain my own personal physical and mental health and provide for all contingencies, which might affect that. It may seem strange to assign this such a high priority, but we have all heard that counter-intuitive bit of advice on airplanes countless times over many years to put on our own masks before tending to the children. The principle is the same.

The physical health of the Carekeeper is very important. At the time of Mona's diagnosis, I thought I was in decent shape. Since then however, I pay significantly more attention to taking care of myself and regularly getting things checked. I also work very hard on improving my efficiency in order to reduce stress.

Maintaining the Carekeeper's personal mental health is equally essential. There is no question that to be able to handle this situation depends on one's adaptability and flexibility in assuming behaviors that are themselves counter-intuitive. I used to assert vehemently that I was never going to adopt bizarre behavior in order to deal with Mona's. I was incorrect.

There are times when the only way to deal with bizarre behavior is by adapting behavior that is even more bizarre although those instances should be as few as possible. To stay mentally healthy, it is a good idea to acknowledge, at least to yourself, that what you are doing need not appear to be very rational to others.

Mona has depended on me more each day, and at the same time, she has become less likely to be able to handle any incidents of my incapacitation. Therefore just as heeding that airborne advice is important on a plane, it is critical to the success of a Carekeeper and so is understanding of the reverse of that equation. One time I had a scary example of this basic logic. In the bargain, I found a weakness in what I had considered a model system for caring for Mona.

One of those common stomach viruses hit me and laid me low. I was in bed and literally too weak to do anything but get from the bed to the bathroom. I knew I was dehydrated and I needed to do something about that. In addition, I knew Mona had an appointment at 9:30 the following morning and I felt that it was not likely I would be able to take her.

Mona was very upset that I was sick, but when I would ask her to get me something to drink or some crackers to eat, she would go down to the kitchen and return with nothing, having forgotten what she was after. Writing it down for her didn't help either.

Finally, I decided to call our son Bob, who lives just a few miles away. When I reached for the telephone, it wasn't there and there was no line in the phone jack on the wall. Obviously, Mona had moved it, but she didn't remember doing that, and worse yet, could not remember where she had put it. I asked her to go down stairs and get the portable phone but I could not make her understand what I wanted, or she couldn't remember when she arrived downstairs. At that point, she was really getting upset.

As soon as I felt better, I tracked down the missing bedroom phone and re-installed it. When I did, I was careful to hide the cord and place the phone on my side of the bed, with the ringer disabled so Mona couldn't hear it. I also put the phone out of sight on the floor under the nightstand.

Ironically, all of this caused me to realize that my incapacitation was Mona's most immediate danger. Therefore, my wellbeing was actually of more pressing concern than hers was. I needed to do something about that. Part of the issue was conceptual, part was procedural, part was operational and part was strategic. All of it is common sense, but I think it is useful to bring it to the attention of those who face what I do.

This obviously is the thrust of the first objective of my plan for Mona's care. I must safeguard and maintain my own personal physical and mental health, providing for all contingencies, which might affect it.

To do that, I needed to heighten my personal perception of my own health and safety and develop a more acute awareness of how our environment affected my new level of activity and the need to care from Mona. I also had to assess, or perhaps have assessed, my level of stress and the possible dangers of that. I had to do those things before anything else.

According to my doctor, I am in excellent health for my age. My heart is sound, my weight, although a little high is constant and manageable, and my blood pressure is enviable. My cholesterol and other lab-measured attributes, except for Triglycerides, are in fine shape. We are working on the Triglycerides. My doctor thinks I should get more exercise, but he has no idea of the number of trips I make up and down stairs monitoring Mona's activities. I would wear out a Stairmaster trying to replicate it.

In the prior five years, I had two highly successful hip replacements. I have no problem getting around now. However, during the months before those two operations and during my recovery from them, I would never have been able to manage Mona's care.

I have great confidence in my Primary Care Physician and he is affiliated with one of the top hospitals in the country. He fulfills my profile of how one should choose a physician. Most people select their own physician in their early twenties. I have always urged my children to do what I did and not look to a friend from high school or college, but to select a doctor who is about fifteen years older. That way, your doctor will be experienced, but well aware of the current technology and he or she should last until you are about fifty. Then, you should pick one who is at least fifteen years younger than you are, for the first two of the same reasons, but also so, you don't outlive them.

My second rationale for choosing my current doctor was that he had a stated special professional interest and Board Certification in both preventive medicine and problems of aging. That seemed to be the correct combination for me and I have been very satisfied with my more than ten-year relationship with him.

Finally, there is a geographical consideration. If one lives in a decent sized metropolitan area, it makes little sense to have to drive more than fifteen minutes to reach a doctor's office. In addition, your doctor should be accessible by phone. If he or she does not return your call the same day, they are either too busy to assure your health or too arrogant for you to tolerate.

Despite my stated criteria, when I realized that Mona's care was going to occupy a large part of my time, I briefly considered the possibility of having the same doctor as she did. It also occurred to me that we might receive more attention as a set, rather than individuals.

I did not make that change for a very important reason. There was a valuable by-product for me in having two doctors. As a practical matter, I was in the presence of Mona's doctor more than my own and not in a passive role. I was communicating to her doctor not only Mona's condition, but her behavior and, therefore, my reactions to it.

Whether Mona's doctor wanted it or not, she was unwittingly observing me in a quite specific manner and I saw that as an opportunity. Since I had developed an excellent rapport with this woman, I had no problem with asking her to provide my doctor with a professional second opinion of my mental and physical well-being.

This strategy has worked well, although the first time it was tried, no doubt responding to my accounts of Mona's behavior and my frustration, her doctor suggested to mine that I might be suffering from mild depression. My doctor, knowing my activity level and general attitude about things, commented that if I were to go on anti-depressant medication, no one would be able to stand me.

I see my doctor every six months, with every other one of those visits, a complete physical. I am rigorously forthcoming about anything unusual although I try to avoid the trivial. I compile a list in between appointments and ask many questions. I follow my doctor's advice as specifically and completely as I can. I stay constantly on the alert for evidence of any changes in stress level.

Because for many years my job made it necessary for me to spend extended periods in the sun, I am prone to develop keratoses on my face. I have them taken care of every six months.

A recent eye examination disclosed early indications of the development of cataracts. That could pose a problem, so we monitor it closely. We will deal with it promptly.

With regard to coping with stress, I am constantly on the alert for ways to simplify my life, combine tasks, reduce their frequency and eliminate some of them. I think of each thing that happens as an opportunity to re-think the way it affects me. An excellent example is laundry.

Our washer and dryer were reaching the end of their useful lives a little before Mona's diagnosis with Alzheimer's Disease. She has always had a thing about laundry, literally doing it every day. For quite a while after her diagnosis, that was something that she could continue to do, and as a result, I paid little or no attention to the process.

Although I was unaware of it, one day the washer stopped during its final rinse cycle and failed to empty the water. Since Mona often would wait until she went downstairs to do the next day's load before moving the washed clothes into the dryer, the next day she just threw the second load on top of the first and re-started the washer.

I'm not sure how many days she did this, but at some point, there was no room for more clothes in the washer. To solve that problem, she moved the huge load of over-soaked, dripping clothes into the dryer. She started the dryer and in short order it overheated and burned out something, which rendered it inoperable.

One would think that the solution was simply to buy a new washer and dryer. However, even though Mona definitely used her washer and dryer more than most people in two person households, I have always believed that having washers and dryers in the home represented one of the worst cost/benefit ratios of any invention in human history.

However, one time, when I was working at Xerox, I was at an off-site, two-week management seminar in New Hampshire. On the middle weekend, we had as a guest lecturer, the world-renowned economist, Herman Kahn. He posed a decision-making situation to us for discussion.

In this situation, a young couple had one car and the woman really wanted them to buy a second one for her personal use. The husband, obviously an economist, calculated how many times and for what purpose she would use this new car.

He then did some investigating and discovered that he could arrange for a chauffer driven car to be available to his wife on five minutes notice any time of the day or night, for substantially less than the cost of them buying even the least expensive new car available and paying for maintenance, insurance and fuel. Kahn posed the question to the group: Given these data, which is the best decision for the husband to make?

The majority of the group, including a much younger me, said he should go for the chauffeur.

Kahn said we were wrong. He should buy the new car for his wife and not the least expensive that he could find. When pressed for a reason to take such counter-intuitive action, Kahn said that we, like the husband, had neglected to factor in the personal cost of the time and the stress of being subjected to the wife's complaining, which he called the bitch factor.

Previously, I would never have mentioned my feelings about the cost/benefit ratio of home laundries and just gone out to buy a washer and dryer. However, now I had a great deal more influence in that decision process and a stake in the outcome.

After obtaining some data on the life expectancy of washers and dryers, researching current prices and making some assumptions about a more reasonable frequency of use, I came to two conclusions: those two appliances would far outlast our need for them; and a reasonable alternative was available at much less cost.

In doing this, I discovered a course of action that would not just simplify my life and would save me money, but it would increase my overall efficiency. However, that was only the beginning.

It was obvious that, with the possible exception of socks and underwear, our wardrobes were sufficient for us to go longer than a week before doing laundry. An investment of a few dollars in socks and underwear could extend that interval to a week and a half or longer.

Now I do the laundry at a Laundromat on Monday of one week, Friday of the second, skip the third and then repeat the pattern. That means that 34 times a year it takes me a little over two and a half hours, including travel time, or about 85 hours per year. Given the wash and dry cycles, Mona's approach would require about 731 hours and 730 trips up and down stairs. The saving of 646 hours is nearly 27 days that I have added to my life, giving me thirteen-month years from this point on. Not bad.

I use three washers and two dryers for a little more than an hour and a half at an annual cost of about $500. It would take more than four years at that rate to recover the purchase cost of a "no frills" new washer and dryer, and I don't have to pay for the hot water or maintenance. However, the savings still don't end.

I pick up coffee and a croissant on my drive to the Laundromat and I read the paper during the wash cycle. During the hour-long drying cycle, I make a run to the nearby supermarket, gas up the car or perform other necessary functions, saving more time.

Here is another example of increasing one's efficiency:

For forty years, we had used the same pharmacy. There was a certain charm in a locally owned business and knowing the owner. Nevertheless, the store has had three other owners in the past few years, and is now part of a national chain.

For several years, the grocery store we frequent has had its own pharmacy, but there hadn't seemed to be a reason to make a change. However, when I considered that it was four miles in one direction to the store, four in the other to the pharmacy, and the pharmacy didn't sell groceries; my course of action was a no-brainer. I also changed branches of the bank I use because the new one, with its free ATM, is on the way.

I try to grocery shop only once a week. To make that a viable proposition, I had to start buying things in larger quantities, which saved me additional money. The once a week routine was not without problems however. It involves freezing meat, fish and poultry and I soon ran into the problem of Mona thawing things arbitrarily. I partially solved that by the out of sight, out of mind method, using the downstairs freezer. To make that work, I just have to be sure that Mona never sees me take anything down to the freezer or bring anything up.

At the store, I keep track of what I spend versus the time it takes me from the car and back, playing a game with myself to increase my spending per minute or, more accurately, reducing the time spent shopping. As a result, I have increased my spending rate to around $2.50 per minute. That means I can make a weekly shopping trip for $100 worth of groceries and supplies in forty minutes from leaving the car in the parking lot to backing out of the spot. That fits the drying cycle at the Laundromat perfectly. I will challenge anyone to maintain that pace, but you had better stay out of my way.

In the interest of economy of energy and increased efficiency, as well as not liking to leave Mona alone much, I try to avoid ever going out for only one reason and I try to minimize the time it takes to do it. I have found that this approach is not only beneficial to me in terms of conserving energy, but that it makes me feel I am winning the task of doing the work that two used to do. It is also somewhat amusing.

I will get into it in more detail in a later chapter, but for now let me just say that Mona and other Alzheimer's victims, often in an effort to be helpful, actually create work to be done, particularly in the area of inefficiency, undoubtedly because they no longer understand that concept. This can become very frustrating and stressful for the Carekeeper.

However, some of that has nothing to do with Alzheimer's. It has to do with style, culture and personal preference. For the first forty-five years of our marriage, and most especially since 1964 when we moved into our home in Pittsford, the house has been Mona's private domain over which she benignly ruled.

Mona did not work full time outside the home. She rarely operated under tight time constraints and efficiency was of lower priority than preference. She kept things where she wanted them and, truth be told, Mona often changed her mind about where that might be.

Mona has also had several other traits. She was an inveterate collector of kitchen gadgets, accumulating most of those known to man. In fact, Mona often had two of some she particularly liked, often in never opened boxes.

Mona has always had great difficulty with throwing things out, even when they were broken, unidentifiable, or parts of something that she had already thrown out. Mona was comfortable with that way of operating, but it had the potential for giving me hypertension or worse.

The effects of Alzheimer's have greatly exacerbated the negative aspects of this way of operating to the point of chaos. It comes in the form of putting things away in strange places, resulting in time consuming, needless and frustrating searches.

It can be in employing unusual processes to accomplish tasks, which themselves create work, such as trying to clean dishes and silverware by just wiping them, thus creating a new task of having to wash these things *before* you use them. It can be thawing things that don't need thawing and freezing things that should not be.

This was no longer an environment conducive to stress-management.

When I first assumed responsibility for preparing all the meals, I was reluctant to make changes in the culture of our kitchen on the theory that it would be stressful to Mona. I soon discovered that I was spending several times longer looking for things than doing anything productive.

As I assumed responsibility for the availability of Mona's clothes, I realized that the same philosophy and culture found in the kitchen was also in play in Mona's dresser and closets. At one point, I estimated that I spent more than half of my time undoing things Mona had done or looking for things. I couldn't do much about the former, but I could and should about the latter.

The Carekeeper cannot take charge of his or her own life and reduce ineffi-ciency and stress without taking at least partial charge of the life of the victim. Laissez-faire is an inoperable concept. I needed help in getting control.

Our daughter, Maryellen, came to the rescue. She came up from Atlanta for several days, five of them days on which Mona was at Day Care. In return for me preparing all the meals, Maryellen accomplished great things in the quest for making me more efficient. She very objectively threw out six large boxes of junk and sent nine large bags of clothes to the Salvation Army.

This is still a work in progress, but things are getting better. There are two components to the burden on the Carekeeper. The first is the extra physical work. The other is the stress. It is part of maintaining the mental health of the Carekeeper to increase efficiency and to reduce the stress. That is critical to a suc-cessful plan for caring for an Alzheimer's victim in the home.

I have found, however, that there are certain tasks that do not yield to this approach, at least not by the application of my levels of skill and effort. Primary among these tasks is keeping the house neat and clean. I have not been able to identify any usable housekeeping skills within my personal capabilities. However, part of the problem may be because there is substantially more to do now.

I am sure there are many people who do not share my feelings about the housekeeping chores not related to the preparation of food. Somehow, when I have spent a long day on errands, appointments and preparing meals, things like dusting, running the vacuum and mopping the kitchen floor lose their priorities. No housekeeper in the world will deny that not keeping on top of things quickly results in an out of control situation.

Actually, although I admit that housekeeping is important, I don't think it is really a care issue. In addition, it is boring to me and I do find it depressing. Of all things related to the current situation, housekeeping is where it is the most obvious to hire someone to help. I needed to do that as soon as possible.

Once again, I am reporting observations rather than hard research data, but my suggestion is that one should make housekeeping decisions carefully and within the context of the Alzheimer's reality. A couple of years before diagnosis, but when it was already very obvious what the problem was, Mona had begun to seriously ignore some housekeeping tasks and do others poorly, and while I was still working from an office outside our home, I hired a cleaning service.

Mona was furious, refusing to let them in the first time they came. The second time, I stayed home until they arrived to manage the situation. Mona seemed to accept that, but as soon as I left, she fired the service. I believe that sub-con-sciously she resented the cleaners and felt they were invading her turf. I think she also interpreted my hiring them as a vote of "no-confidence" in her ability to function as fully as she once had. Recently, when I have needed the service, I have had them come when Mona is not at home and leave before she returns.

Cleaning services are expensive and the rates they charge are double that of an independent. The problem is that it is difficult to find a responsible independent in many areas and they enjoy a sellers market.

I believe that a Carekeeper, particularly if male, with a little effort, patience and the appearance of basic incompetence in the matter, can find a relatively inexpensive solution to the housekeeping problem without hiring a service. The impression of incompetence is critical.

The presence of an outsider in the house can be disturbing to the victim. The fact that it is on a regular basis doesn't help, since they no longer comprehend routine. Victims often do not feel they are impaired. However, since the skill involved to do the housekeeping yourself is modest and the victim does not really know or care that your time is valuable; they feel you should just do it. The secret lies in finding a reasonable middle ground.

I found a competent, independent professional cleaning person who is very adept at doing a big job in a relatively short time. I bring her in for major cleaning projects. Then I try to keep up as best I can without making it a crusade. When I begin to see that I am really losing the battle, I bring back the professional to help me.

All of these things and others make it possible for me to do the things that I have to do more efficiently and with less expenditure of energy and time, but they do not necessarily promote better mental health. That requires a completely different approach and a certain amount of dedication.

I am sure that means that no one approach will suit everyone. I can only tell you what seems to be working for me.

First, with my office, I established a space that is solely mine. It is more than an office. It is a retreat and a refuge. However, from that position I can monitor by sound and smell, virtually everything that is going on in the house, aided and abetted by an alert dog that is devoted to Mona and will bark only when I can be sure that something warrants my presence and attention.

Secondly, I try to communicate every aspect of Mona's condition and other matters of common interest to our children, adult grandchildren, all their spouses and significant others. This gives me peace of mind that in an emergency they could step in without missing a beat.

Thirdly, I have a large array of projects, which have nothing to do with my primary job of Carekeeper or the management of our affairs. They include maintaining a regular and lively e-mail correspondence with as many people as possible and continually looking for new people to add. I also monitor and contribute to an Internet Forum for people who were in college with me whether we were friends or not and I pursue an avocation of being a news junkie, keeping up with a broad range of current events. However, providing the most stimulation and enjoyment, I try to write for several hours every day.

The writing has been the most helpful because it challenges my mind the most. This book is a product of that effort. Before undertaking this one, I wrote a book called "The Compliant, Curious & Critical Catholic". I have finished the first twenty-five years of a book of personal remembrances and stories called "Decades". I am working on a tongue in cheek look at public policy called "Please Don't Call Me a Liberal … It Makes Us Both Sound Silly". Moreover, I have some other projects in mind, including a novel about a group of mobsters operating out of an assisted living facility.

Finally, I am constantly looking for things to keep my mind active. I take all the quizzes I come across on the Internet, especially those about which I know little or nothing. I have found that I get about 50% on the latter, which apparently means that a passing score is being sure of only about 25% of your answers and that seems to be about the same as with most things in life.

Because of all these things, on balance I think I am doing okay. The most important thing is to achieve balance and that is different for each person.

It is very important to recognize that there is no way for the Carekeeper to go through this ordeal unscathed. Please don't feel for a moment that you should. This is part of the human experience. It is what makes us worthwhile. The only real compensation comes in the knowledge that you have done as well as you could, for as long as is necessary.

Sure, you can feel a little sorry for yourself, but get over it. I know that I am already a very different person than I used to be, but strange as it may seem, I think I may be a better one. Maybe I am not really better but certainly, I have not become worse. Well, maybe a little worse in one respect.

Let's deal with that downside first.

The loss of my major conversation partner after nearly fifty years has made me different, especially in the last few years. I crave verbal interaction, and when there is a situation in which I have an opportunity, I babble. I am an equal opportunity babbler. I babble to anyone, whether family, friends or clerks in a store.

Pity the poor person who unwittingly asks me a simple question. Unfortunately, the babble often seems to me in retrospect to be somewhat self-centered. I really hate that and am working hard at changing it.

On the plus side, I have developed a new set of heroes. I have four good friends who lost their wives to terrible diseases after years of suffering, and another who has been going through that for many years. Two of them took over and raised their children. Those are the real heroes. By comparison, my lot is easy.

CHAPTER 4

▼

THE TEAM IS LARGER THAN IT LOOKS IN THE MIRROR

The second interim goal in my plan to serve as Mona's Carekeeper was to develop an effective support team. This is far more than writing down an address and phone list of people with whom one should keep in touch. I needed to develop and maintain constant communication with a functional support system of medical personnel, relatives and friends, services, systems and procedures.

A longer-term key element is the designation of a Deputy Carekeeper who is fully cognizant of everything going on and can take over completely in an emergency for an extended period. Implicit in that is a level of communication, which is unusual even in families.

Once again, there is no magic way to undertake either of these tasks and I can only share my thought process and approach.

Fortunately, this system need not be labor intensive in the sense of needing a large number of people involved, particularly at the outset. The secret is to attempt to make at least some of the disparate elements of your life work together, producing synergy. It is all about efficiency and a philosophy of simultaneously reducing the effort required, while producing the desired results.

Both the personal circumstances of the potential Carekeeper, and his or her psychological makeup, are factors of viability for the job, and by extension, the breadth and depth of that job. Clearly, that varies with the individual, but they all need the continual support of others to make up for their deficiencies.

Carekeepers may appear on the surface to be heroic, but truth be told, for the most part their heroism is reluctant. The same is true for the other members of the team whether they are caregivers, caretakers or something else entirely. They are just doing their best to do what needs doing. No one really wants these jobs.

In my case, I was in good health and had the desire to be deeply involved in Mona's health, safety and quality of life. Therefore, at least at the outset, I didn't need much day-to-day assistance, except in the case of emergencies. I did however, need to identify those who I might need in the future or sooner if the situation were to change, even if that meant to merely keep them fully aware of the situation on a continual basis.

The most important aspect of the selection of the support team is that one doesn't settle for mediocrity. Both the Carekeeper and the Alzheimer's victim must depend on everyone doing his or her job. If someone is not up to the task, pass him or her up or involve him or her in another, less critical way. Do that regardless of what their relationship is with you or the victim.

Sometimes that means passing up family members, but family loyalty cannot affect your judgment. Your first loyalty is to the victim. You need the best there is. If you don't have that, you will end up doing both your job and his or hers.

In putting together the team, it is only natural to look to one's family and friends for support, but that not always practical. For example, Mona and I have three married children and four adult grandchildren. With spouses and significant others, that is a cadre of fourteen people. All fourteen of them are realistic about the situation, intensely interested and supportive. Not one of those fourteen would refuse for an instant to do whatever they could do for Mona or to help me. They would be insulted if anyone were to suggest otherwise. However, none of them is in a position to be a regular Carekeeper.

Twelve of those fourteen lead their lives from more than 300 to nearly 3,000 miles away. For them to be physically involved on a regular basis is obviously impractical. Fortunately, the other two are less than six miles away and equally willing. However, they both work and have three teenage daughters, so their regular, scheduled involvement is equally impractical, although they are always available in an emergency.

Consequently, there is no formal Deputy Carekeeper, sufficiently acquainted with the details of Mona's routine to take over. It is my responsibility to find one and I need to do something about that. The answer clearly is better communications and I suspect that if I can solve that issue, it will be beneficial to all members of the team, not just those who are local. This is a priority item and I will address it later in this chapter.

I do maintain regular telephone and e-mail contact with all seven families. In addition, I send out an e-mail report of Mona's mental and physical health, which includes my personal observations. By definition, this is anecdotal in nature, but I try to minimize the trivial. I do this because they have every right to know everything about Mona's condition. I also do not want them to be shocked when they see her, because subtle changes constantly occur.

All of these families remain in regular contact with Mona by phone and that is important for them as well as for her. It prepares them for the times when they do see her and eases their distress with her deterioration. Sometimes it is confusing to Mona, but her appreciation of the contact far outweighs that.

I need to upgrade significantly these communications in a creative way. Ironically, this may have an unplanned benefit. The big losers from Mona's disease are the younger grandchildren and now the great-grandchildren. The gathering of memories and shared experiences ended abruptly and will always remain unfinished for the former and the latter will never have that opportunity. Perhaps reading the communications within the support team will help fill that need. So will this book.

There is another important reason to keep one's family fully informed of the victim's condition from the outset, although thankfully, it does not affect us. There is a form of Alzheimer's Disease, called Early Onset Alzheimer's, which afflicts its victims in their late forties or early fifties. This is usually an inherited, genetic strain, which puts children and siblings at risk.

As with many diseases, early detection is very important. This is especially true with Early Onset Alzheimer's, since the few medications available appear to be most effective if taken even before symptoms appear.

Let us now discuss what I consider the essential elements of an initial Carekeeper's Support Team. Like a professional football team, there are three parts: Offense, Defense and Special Teams. To extend the analogy, without overstating it, the Carekeeper functions not only as Head Coach but also as General Manager.

The first element is the Offense. It may seem obvious to say so, but there are some subtleties here and I have some suggestions, which I found helpful.

Every good coach knows he should always avoid a quarterback controversy. The victim's Primary Care Physician must be assured that he or she is the quarterback and the one with whom you discuss every aspect of the care. Otherwise, they may not accept that full responsibility. However, that does not mean that the Coach (Carekeeper) need not be fully knowledgeable of every aspect of the victim's condition and treatment.

Mona's Primary Care Physician is an outstanding woman and we have an excellent rapport. If she tells me something that needs doing, I get it done. Conversely, if I express a concern, she knows that I don't do that lightly and investigates it thoroughly.

Aside from having severe Alzheimer's Disease, Mona's overall physical health is excellent. She takes a fair number of medications, but her Primary Care Physician, whom she visits on four-month intervals, carefully monitors them.

The second most important member of the Offense is the Clinical Psychiatrist who tracks the progression (I say regression) of Alzheimer's. It is important to realize that it would be easy for one of two scenarios to develop, both undesirable. In the first, the victim essentially has two Primary Care Physicians, one for his or her brain and the other for everything else. In the second scenario, the Clinical Psychiatrist effectively disappears.

The latter is easy to understand, since there is no specific treatment requiring his or her constant attention. In addition, such doctors are primarily researchers and to some degree, many are uncomfortable with regular patient contact, perhaps because the victim always gets worse.

The Psychiatrist should be kept involved to the greatest possible degree. He or she is the Primary Care Physician's eyes and ears regarding Alzheimer's, and to extend the analogy acts like a Quarterback Coach. It is important to keep him or her involved through regular appointments. Once again, Mona was very fortunate, relatively speaking. The Clinical Psychiatrist who made her initial diagnosis was Dr. Pierre Tariot and he is an internationally known expert on Alzheimer's.

Through Dr. Tariot, Mona participated in a two-year clinical trial, which I will discuss later, that kept Tariot and his staff involved in her observation, if not her care. The trial is complete and Dr. Tariot has now moved on to a similar position in Arizona.

The trick is to give the Psychiatrist some motivation to remain involved. As in any other human relationship, that is easier if you give them something they need or want. Clinical trials are the perfect vehicle. I will say much more about this in Chapter Six.

Since Mona is in very good physical health, she has only occasional needs for other medical professionals other than her designated Gynecologist, but when and if she does, I always insist on the same protocol. Everyone takes direction from the quarterback, her Primary Care Physician, and she controls the prescription and administration of all medication.

I have told Mona's Primary Care Physician that it is her job to assure that Mona dies of Alzheimer's Disease. Obviously, that statement is somewhat facetious, but it also is accurate.

The protocol is simple. Her Primary Care Physician, in the form of consultations, which require written reports, manages all visits to all medical professionals for examination or testing. The PCP reviews and writes any recommended prescriptions.

We agree that periodically the PCP will ask for a consulting visit to the Clinical Psychiatrist for evaluation. I feel that is sufficient.

In addition, I insist on being physically present in the examining room for all visits to every medical professional and feel completely free to ask any question which comes to mind, whenever it does. That way I serve as the eyes and ears of the PCP and I feel competent to make my own comments on the written reports of these consulting professionals.

In a later chapter, I will deal with additional members of our Offensive Unit who, along with those in our Defensive Unit, also play on Special Teams. I am very comfortable with that arrangement.

Extending the football analogy, our Defensive Unit is equally important and the Head Coach/Carekeeper functions as the Defensive Coordinator. The Unit involves the fourteen adult members of our immediate family, augmented over time as others come of age. They represent varying levels of availability, but the same degree of interest and commitment.

At present, their involvement is advisory and supportive, but that will change. Our daughter, Maryellen, who lives in Georgia, currently has the most flexibility since her children are older and all married. If needed, she could function as Carekeeper for a week or two. She is also available for special projects, such as major makeovers of Mona's wardrobe.

Alzheimer's is a disease of patience and waiting and loneliness. The fact of the matter is that one cannot shorten or lengthen the duration and intensity of those things by additional participation. My greatest challenge with the Defense Unit is to keep them all involved, fully informed and highly motivated about our situation. I intend to do that.

It would be natural at this point for a reader to ask about the participation of family members of Mona's and my generation. We each had one sister and no brothers. Both lived ninety miles away in the Syracuse area. Sadly, my sister died in early 2001. I try to keep Mona's sister fully informed about specific details.

Obviously, when a person has Alzheimer's Disease, many people, friends and family alike are affected and reactions are often mixed and sometimes surprising. Once again, other people's experiences may be quite different from mine. However, I suspect that the same reactions occur, but they just come from different people.

Those of us of "Alzheimer's Age" are enlightened only to the extent to which we may have had to deal with the disease in our parents. Our parents were generally secretive about such things and spoke of them in hushed tones.

I am sure that with our generation, a feeling of unease exists about the actual diagnosis of Alzheimer's Disease as the result of the reaction of our parents to it or as they called it, "hardening of the arteries". In their day, life expectancy was such that fewer people became victims of Alzheimer's. There also was a certain stigma attached to people who suffered any kind of Dementia, equating it to insanity and some sociopathic disorders. They often hid their relatives who were afflicted.

I certainly do not feel that suffering from Alzheimer's is any disgrace and I suspect that if asked most of my peers would agree with that assessment. However, many of them act uncomfortable in Mona's presence or as if they just want to ignore what has happened to her even to the point of saying the obviously incorrect, "she seems better".

Probably that is because the disease is so debilitating and since it seems related to the aging process, it therefore appears to be everyone's inevitable fate. It is, I suppose, natural for them to feel that way around the victim, regardless of their prior relationship.

I also believe that this feeling is significantly greater in the siblings of the Alzheimer's victim. They are fearful that they are looking at the way they may soon be. However, beyond that they are often in sufficient denial that they believe since they have so many more shared memories, for so many more years, that they may be able to evoke the one memory which will sweep the clouds away in the way we all have often seen happen in old movies.

Obviously, since I haven't researched this subject, that statement is merely an observation of the reaction and behavior of Mona's sister. Certainly, not all people react similarly and to some degree my observations may be inaccurate or unfair. Nevertheless, they do provide a good level of empirical data for consideration.

Mona's sister is five years younger and, as adults, they have always been close. It was difficult for her to accept Mona's diagnosis, perhaps because of the fear that it might some day also be hers.

Moreover, I have always had the sense that she was not entirely convinced that my assessment of the situation was accurate. That is completely understandable. She talks to Mona at least once a week. She lives just an hour and a half away, and since both she and her husband are retired, every few weeks they drive up and we all go out to lunch.

Nonetheless, in the years since Mona's diagnosis, she has never once suggested that Mona visit her, even for a few days. In fact, privately to other family members, she has said that she could not handle that.

Their phone chats have become briefer and briefer and when they are together, the conversation is more like an interview, with Mona's sister asking question after question to test what Mona can remember or perhaps to stimulate her memory. The result is upsetting to both of them and I have taken to cutting off the questions almost as soon as they begin, but the pattern repeats at the next opportunity. I hope her sister understands that.

This behavior also has some elements of second-guessing; so I do not encourage participation in any decision-making. However, I do keep her informed of Mona's condition and I sugar coat nothing.

Friends are another matter.

I was somewhat prepared for their reaction, based on my experience at the time in late December of 1993 when Mona was in the hospital and the rehab program would not accept her because of her memory loss. Then I learned that they were about to discharge Mona and that I had to meet with the Social Worker as soon as possible.

The Social Worker's opinion was that I could not provide adequate care and Mona could not go home. Since Mona's insurance would no longer cover her care in the hospital, if she stayed there, we would be liable for the expense.

I called everyone I thought could help me get her in to a Nursing Home on at least a temporary basis. Some were doctors, some lawyers, some Board members of Nursing Homes. Their response no doubt at least partly because it was a busy Christmas Eve, was lukewarm at best, but they all promised to get back to me. None ever did.

On the day after Christmas, in an effort to buy her time to negotiate further with the rehab facility, her Primary Care Physician, probably contrary to the hospital rules, had Mona transferred to the Psychiatric Floor. Fortunately, she was only there for ten days before they finally accepted her for rehab. However, visiting a terrified Mona on the Psychiatric Floor each day, for what seemed an eternity, was an experience I will not forget.

I have felt from the outset that Mona should continue to participate in life for as long as possible and that people should accept her, as they would if she were deaf, blind or crippled. In her case, she responds very well to people, leaving nearly all who see her only occasionally believing that she is far better than she really is.

I speak freely and candidly about her condition. In fact, this book evolved from a fourteen-page update on her condition, which I wrote and distributed a few years ago to friends and relatives who hadn't seen Mona for a while, but would be attending our eldest granddaughter's wedding.

I did that so that they would feel comfortable and would greet and interact with Mona on her terms. People responded well and several encouraged me to write more. I am doing so, hoping that it will lead to better understanding of a disease which will soon affect many more families.

When we are in a store or a restaurant or in any situation involving an interaction with Mona, I try subtly to make the other person aware of her condition. Usually, they make an effort to treat her with kindness and respect and seem to appreciate that I informed them.

One day, while reading a newspaper, I came across a suggestion from the Carekeeper of an Alzheimer's victim. He said that he had business cards made, describing his wife's situation, which he handed to waiters, clerks and anyone else they encountered. I thought that was brilliant and stole the idea. Mine reads:

> *My Name Is Bob Betterton*
> *And My Wife Is Mona*
> *Unfortunately, Mona suffers from advanced Alzheimer's Disease.*
> *She is very social and enjoys personal interaction.*
> *Please feel free to deal with her in that way.*
> *I will handle any decisions, which may be required,*
> *including purchases and ordering meals.*
> *Thank you for your understanding.*

Although that helps with strangers, I have been surprised and somewhat disappointed at the reluctance of people who I have considered her good friends, to take any initiative to contact either Mona directly, or me about her. I am not sure I understand that, because these are good people. Consider the following two examples among many I could cite.

Mona had a good friend who moved to Pittsford nearly forty years ago, shortly after we did. When she moved here, she didn't drive and for months, Mona chauffeured her all over the place as she became familiar with the area and settled her home. Mona never once complained about doing that and even drove the woman to take her driving test. The two had become very close friends.

That friendship continued for many years. Mona and her friend have always gone to the same hairdresser and for many years, they scheduled their appointments one after the other, spending the full time in conversation. Then they would go to lunch.

During the time in which Mona was in the hospital for alcoholism, her friend visited her several times. However, as Mona began to have more and more memory problems, their contacts became less frequent and finally stopped.

When the doctor diagnosed Mona with Alzheimer's, I called to tell her friend. They still go to the same hairdresser and it would be an easy thing for Mona's friend to schedule their appointments back to back, the way they used to do, at least once and a while. She could pick Mona up and they could have lunch. Mona would like that. However, it has never happened.

Recently a mutual friend died and Mona and I went to the funeral. As luck would have it, Mona's friend arrived at the church at the same time we did. She asked if she could sit with us and we readily agreed. It appeared to me that she deliberately arranged it so that she did not sit next to Mona, but that I was between them.

Another close friend of Mona's has always been solicitous about Mona's condition, whenever I run into her. I called her about Mona's Alzheimer's diagnosis. She wanted to know what she could do and asked if she could call Mona. When I said that would be great, she asked if she could stop by or if she could take Mona to lunch some day. I said she should feel free to do that anytime.

That woman lives about a quarter of a mile from us. My conversation with her was more than three years ago. She has never called. I feel sorry for both her and Mona. Sadly, these things happened while Mona was still conscious of their neglect. She mentioned it often, puzzled at why they didn't seem to care.

I have found that one should not expect much help from old friends or associates. However, I do not intend that for many as criticism and it isn't because they are unwilling. They can do little at arm's length. With this disease, they don't need to give blood. They can't administer therapy. No one need do that sort of thing.

However, I obviously did not want any of these people to be on the team, although some in my situation do not have a family like mine on whom they can rely. However, that is not why I have brought it up. It is just sad that these friends and others are no longer a part of Mona's life. Both they and others have lost something very valuable and difficult to replace. Friendship.

In the early stages when this happens, the victim feels abandoned. It is a natural thing for them to expect that friends and family will call or visit. Nevertheless, that becomes doubly heartbreaking and a seemingly useless effort when those calls and the visits <u>are</u> made, but not remembered and go unappreciated. That still is not a valid reason for not doing it.

Eventually the victim forgets his or her friend. I suppose that in the great cosmos, that makes them even, because the friend remembers that Mona forgot her.

That is enough dwelling on things one cannot affect. Let's get back to the Carekeeper's support team and operational setup.

As I wrote this, Mona's care requirements are of two types: those things that she used to do for the two of us, and those that she used to be able to do.

We have already discussed the things she used to do for the two of us, such as shopping, cooking, laundry and housekeeping. I have assumed responsibility for all of those, and if I do say so myself, I do an excellent job of all but the last.

The things that she used to do for herself, but is no longer able to do, are maintaining her own schedule, driving a car, going to activities outside the home by herself and managing money. There also is managing her wardrobe in terms of selecting what to wear, the sequence of dressing, managing her personal hygiene in terms of remembering to shower, shampoo and brush her teeth and putting things in their proper place.

I have pretty much taken over these things, and except for the last item, Mona has quietly acquiesced. She continues to try constantly to put things in their proper place. However, she rarely if ever, remembers where that is.

The caregivers or caretakers on the team can do many things to help. However, remember that no matter who is helping, there is only one <u>Carekeeper</u>. It is very useful to have thought through the nature of each task so that you only delegate caretaker or caregiver tasks to the team members. It is also critical for you to understand what they offer when someone tells you that they would like to help or to "give you a hand". Accept all offers, especially early on, so that you can assess the level of support you really have.

Most important of all, learn to distinguish between commiseration and assistance. There is a time and a place for both and, if you don't make the distinction, neither will be available to you when you need them the most. The funny thing is that although you need a certain and relatively constant level of commiseration, your need for real assistance will increase. However, there will always be more commiseraters available than real assisters. That can become a problem.

Set some ground rules and let them help you distinguish between those two kinds of need. If you want commiseration, go have a beer with a friend and talk, even if that requires assistance in the form of someone to be with the victim. Don't mix the two.

If one of your children or grandchildren comes over to "help you out" make them really do it and go have that beer with someone else, or just go sit in the park with the sun on your face. Sitting around, sharing anecdotes about the victim's deteriorating condition seems sometimes to be a viable activity, but usually it makes everyone depressed, and worse yet, could lead the person you may need to help you some day, to want to avoid that feeling of depression.

Sound advice is "don't expect much and you will not be disappointed", although that is not meant as criticism. Equally sound advice is "never assume you really know what people are willing to do". The care of an Alzheimer's victim is burdensome and relentless. It also never gets easier.

The intent here is not to inflict guilt, but to build an effective team. The size and the makeup of that team depend on the situation, and that situation is likely to change over time.

Carekeeping is a full-time job and there is no way to divide it up efficiently. However, in Mona's current state, and probably until she must have skilled care, Caretaking is not even a demanding part time job and its real need is far too random to be scheduled. For the most part, the Carekeeper must absorb the Caretaker functions. That can be exhausting.

Throughout the time I was making these adjustments in my life in order to accommodate Mona's needs, there remained the reality of having no Deputy Carekeeper in case of my extended absence or incapacitation. My temporary solution is "The Mona Book". This approach will be no surprise to those who know me well. They will no doubt, react with "he's doing that thing again".

Ironically, that is the truth. In 1954, when I was a newly commissioned Ensign in the Navy I was sent to a highly secure Navy installation in Washington, DC. Since I did not yet have the required clearance for a regular assignment, I was in a group of several junior officers, who on a rotating basis manned the Quarterdeck twenty-four hours a day, seven days a weeks.

This amounted to being a highly educated, and for the Navy, highly paid receptionist, with an astounding collection of randomly occurring mundane, brainless and routine tasks, any one of which, if not handled correctly, could result in a Court Martial. To pass the time, I put together a completely unofficial "What To Do If … Manual". I have been doing the same thing for more than fifty years.

"The Mona Book" is a white loose-leaf binder with everything I can think of that one would have to know about keeping Mona's care. It is an on-going, ever-changing, work in progress.

Please note that there is another very important, ex-officio member of the support group and ad hoc captain of Special Teams, Tipper. In many ways, large and small, one of the best things Mona has going for her is her dog.

Tipper is a red and white, pure bred Border Collie. Our daughter, Maryellen, gave her to Mona over my vigorous objections, just about the time that her worsening Alzheimer's was becoming obvious. I was very wrong in my assessment of the introduction of the dog into our lives.

Mona was even more opposed to having another dog in the house than I was, so Tipper's future was far from secure. We had "been there and done that". For more than forty years, we had owned and loved a distinguished succession of Beagles. I knew that a Beagle just wouldn't work in this situation. However, we did not know about Border Collies, trained for centuries to care for herds of sheep, regardless of what the danger or the weather.

Perhaps other breeds would do well in this situation, but I think Tipper is exceptional. The manual says Border Collies are happiest when they have a job. Tipper immediately sensed that her job is Mona. Not only does Tipper provide Mona with someone to care for, feed and even talk to, she senses Mona's every mood and responds.

If Mona goes silent because she is sad that she can't remember something, Tipper is at her side, demanding that Mona pet her. If Mona rejects her, she lays down at Mona's feet ready whenever needed.

If Tipper is outside and hears Mona's voice, she wants to come in. If she is in and Mona goes out into the yard or garage, Tipper immediately bounds up the stairs to search me out and she won't take no for an answer until I go and check out the situation. Mona's life would be much less without Tipper. It is a beautiful thing to watch.

Even if there has never been a dog in your home, I would definitely recommend trying to bring a Border Collie like Tipper into an Alzheimer's household. It is good for all involved, Carekeeper as well as the victim and the dog.

CHAPTER 5

▼

MAINTAINING LIFESTYLES

Shortly after Mona's diagnosis, but with no reference to Alzheimer's she began to work into our daily conversation a statement that she loved our home and never wanted to move. Although I knew that was probably not a practical scenario, I became determined to try to honor that preference at least until she would not perceive that I hadn't.

It has long been my personal observation and now is widely accepted even by medical professionals that if you force people to change their residence as the result of illness the move itself often accelerates the deterioration of their condition. I did not want the same thing that happened to my mother to happen to Mona.

Following the death of my father, my mother went through an extended period of profound grief with attendant depression. She had lived alone for over ten years in a two-story house and although she was physically very healthy and did not suffer Dementia, when she reached her mid-eighties my sister and I became concerned about her situation.

Ultimately, we convinced my mother to move into a Senior Living Facility. At first, she lived in the Independent Living section and was quite self-sufficient. I was very much in favor of this move, but in retrospect, I believe that leaving her familiar surroundings and giving up the related feeling of independence took a serious toll. Her physical, mental and emotional condition declined rapidly.

Within a month or so after moving in she moved into Assisted Living and before too much longer, she required increasingly higher levels of care. In my opinion, at least with my mother that residence change exacerbated her decline. It made her or at least encouraged her to give up.

In Mona's case, from the outset, keeping her at home for some extended period seemed an achievable goal. Unlike some Alzheimer's victims, at the time of her diagnosis Mona was not wanderer, nor had she shown any violent behavior. She could dress herself, feed herself, take care of her personal needs and operate the TV. She definitely did not require constant supervision. That is not to say, however, that she did not require attention.

Mona has only lived in four places in her entire life. She has lived 55% of her life in our current home, 33% in that of her parents and only 12% in the combined other two. I became determined that there must be extraordinary reasons for Mona to move again, but cognizant that they will inevitably occur.

Both my third and fourth Interim Goals address the objective of allowing Mona to stay at home for as long as possible. The third is to provide a safe and secure environment in our home for Mona, so that the environment is never an issue in determining where she may or may not live. The fourth is to provide Mona a lifestyle, which includes as much freedom as possible to do what she wants to do, consistent with her health and safety. These objectives are closely related and this chapter will cover the way we have dealt with both.

My approach has been, as with so much else at the same time, largely intuitive but carefully considered. However, I have learned over time that some aspects of our plan are rather revolutionary and some people cautioned me several times against saying much about them to Mona's doctors or, God forbid, a social worker. It is too late for that, but I think it is silly anyway. Mona thrives in and is happy with the environment we have established and she shows signs of continuing in that mode.

My observation, confirmed by a number of Alzheimer's experts and Carekeepers such as I am is that few Alzheimer's victims are the same at least until they reach the advanced severe stage. Our approach to Mona's care may be yet another example that standardized care is not always the most effective or humane.

Moreover, once again this approach is possible in our circumstances and depends on the fact that I am healthy and understand the need for strategy and planning. The result is that I can do most of it myself. It also is easier for me to do it because these are familiar surroundings for me as well.

I am generally able to work my schedule around Mona's needs. That gets tricky some times, but I have found that if I tell people why I can't do something at a specific time they usually are very willing to accommodate me.

In other words, there were no inherent reasons why I could not at least for the immediate future care for Mona at home under reasonable environmental conditions. Deciding on and if necessary making changes in our environmental conditions was the next project.

Let us begin with the physical aspects of our home and neighborhood. Like most of the early settlers, we built our home in the early sixties. The design of the tract is rather random and the folklore of the residents has it that the only way one can find one's way out to the main road is by accident. That said the main road is more than a quarter of a mile away and Mona has never been a walker.

Our house is a two-story classic center entrance, four-bedroom Colonial of 2,400 square feet, located on a third of an acre. The large back yard is completely fenced, not because of Mona, but because we have a dog and an enforced leash law.

The kitchen and family room, where the only downstairs TV is located, are contiguous across two-thirds of the back of the house, and a pleasant, enclosed back porch opens off the family room. From the porch, one can exit to the patio and the fenced back yard.

Our bedroom runs the depth of the house, above the living room. It is large, with a walk-in closet, a private bath and the only other TV. It is not immediately adjacent to the stairs. My office is in another bedroom at the rear on the other side of the house, over the kitchen and at the top of the stairway. I have a keen sense of both hearing and smell, from that position and with the door open I can easily monitor everything that is going on in the house. Since my office is located over the kitchen and it is next to the garage I can easily hear all outside doors opening and closing.

We cook with electricity, so there is no danger from escaping gas or fire unless there is something flammable in a pan on an active burner. Although Mona had been an accomplished cook, I began doing most of the cooking even before her diagnosis. Therefore, the usual dangers associated with the kitchen are virtually non-existent.

There did not seem to be any physical changes required immediately, but there were certain things we modified particularly in the area of physical safety. From the outset, although Mona had not shown any wandering tendencies, I had to be conscious of that eventuality and alert to its development, without suggesting it to her.

My mother used to say, "Don't put beans up your nose"! That was a reference to a story about an overprotective mother who, when leaving her child alone made that admonition.

Of course, the child had never previously considered putting beans up his nose and didn't even know where his mother kept the beans, but she had prompted his curiosity about something he had never tried and sounded like fun. Sure enough, when his mother returned he had found the beans and had inserted several in each nostril to his unbridled amusement.

Mindful of that story, I did not investigate the installation of digital password and alarm protected door locks or notify the Sheriff's Office of the presence of an Alzheimer's victim in our house. I also didn't enroll Mona in the Safe Home program touted by the Alzheimer's Association.

While I am at it, I would like to say something about the Safe Home program, which provides identity bracelets to the victim and some valuable information for the Carekeeper. In my opinion, this is a perfect example of an excellent idea suffering from poor implementation.

According to the Alzheimer's Association statistics, 60% of all Alzheimer's victims will eventually wander. They provide excellent information regarding who is at risk, what may prompt them to wander, when they are most likely to do it and how to make it difficult for them to escape the home. For a fee of $40, they also provide several different types of identification, including a bracelet for the victim to wear; and they enroll them in a database, which is accessible by law enforcement.

The problem is that it is nearly as difficult to identify a wandering Alzheimer's victim as to identify a terrorist. Before attending my first informational seminar, I had never heard of the Safe Home program and for most of the others attending that was the case. None of the medical professionals had mentioned it and it was not included in any of the material sent me, or if it were, it was not an identified priority item for consideration.

As a test, try asking your friends and family what they would do if they encountered a confused, elderly person wandering down the street. Ask a policeman if you know one. I doubt that very many would say that you should look for a bracelet.

That being said as soon as Mona displays any tendency to wander, I would enroll her in the program. I just don't want to suggest that she "not put beans up her nose". I will also hope that if she gets out of my sight whoever sees her has heard of Safe Home and will look for a bracelet.

The stairs to the second floor have thus far not appeared to present a danger. Mona is steady on her feet and has always used the railing when ascending or descending on her very frequent daily trips.

The stairs to the basement are a bit more dangerous because they are slightly steeper and there is no railing on one side. However, since Mona stopped doing the laundry and fixing meals, she has no reason to go into the basement. I don't think she has been down there in months.

In the meantime, my precautions consist of being alert to doors opening and closing as well as checking on why they are. This is slightly more difficult in the summer.

I had some concern regarding the safeguarding of valuables. In approaching that issue, one should remember that with an Alzheimer's victim, out of sight is definitely out of mind, with no pun intended.

There are a modest number of collectibles in our house and I have tried to move the more fragile items out of harm's way, bringing some into my office where I can monitor Mona's admiring of them. However, the contents of the china cabinet merit vigilance. A crystal wine glass has been broken, but in a normal accident. There may come a time when locks are considered.

On a couple of occasions, I have had to rescue a sterling silver dinner knife that she was about to use as a screwdriver, but that generally seems a small problem.

I am beginning to suspect that because Mona is not doing any cooking at all, she has forgotten how to operate the stove. I know that to be true of the microwave. The main problem is with her randomly adjusting temperature and timer settings for the stove, microwave and crockpot. Mona also seems to have developed a propensity for freezing things, which should not be frozen, thawing things that should not be, and putting things away in strange places.

Food is probably the most at-risk commodity in our house. Other than that in my opinion, we have established a safe and comfortable environment in which Mona can live. Within it, Mona has a lifestyle, which simultaneously recognizes her needs and challenges her abilities. She has few constraints and seems to thrive under this approach.

I will discuss the idiosyncrasies of Mona's behavior and the ways in which I deal with them in Chapter Seven. In this chapter, I will continue to address just the underlying philosophy of my attitude toward Mona's care. I think I describe that accurately as tightly monitored permissiveness. For the most part, she has significant freedom.

On Mondays, Wednesdays and Fridays, Mona attends an adult day care program and the diver picks her up around 9:30 AM. I have learned from experience that the shorter the time between being ready to go and actually leaving, the better.

Therefore, I wake her at a little before nine with her medications in one hand and a glass of water in the other. She never wants to get up so to get her moving I must resort to blatant chicanery. I will discuss her sleep patterns in a later chapter because I think that is an important and interesting subject.

I present Mona with the medications and water with a slight sense of urgency, which gets her attention and before Mona can suggest otherwise I tell her she has to sit on the edge of the bed so I won't spill the water on her. As soon as she downs the medications and the water, I take both of her hands and playfully pull her to her feet rewarding her with a hug when she does as I direct.

Usually, with a bit of urgency in her voice Mona says she has to go to the toilet. I make the bed while she is in the bathroom washing her face and brushing her teeth. That precludes her option of climbing back in. I also lay out her clothes for the day.

Mona dresses herself including double tying the laces of her sneakers and brushing her own hair. Sometimes I have to do a little repair work on the back of her hair but overall she does a good job. I make sure Mona has her glasses and then she is ready to go.

Tuesday and Thursday mornings a Home Health Aide visits for an hour, arriving about 8:15 AM. She is there to help Mona take a shower and if time and weather permit, they take a walk.

Once again, we have learned that Mona is more cooperative when she awakes and receives immediate direction so the routine is the same. However, I leave them alone as soon as I have given Mona the medications and the water. That transfer of control works like a charm.

Once the Aide leaves, unless she has an appointment Mona is on her own. She usually occupies her day with letting Tipper in and out and keeping her food and water dishes full, trying to read the paper, working on "Find the Word" puzzles, watching TV, and snacking. She also gets considerable exercise by coming upstairs to show or tell me things. It is common for her to make fifteen or more round trips on the stairs in the course of the day.

If I smell something cooking, I immediately investigate. I never leave the kitchen while I am cooking something on the surface of the stove. If I am cooking something in the oven or a slow cooker, I check often to make sure that the timer and temperature have not changed.

Mona was a largely self-taught, excellent cook. For many years she taught cooking techniques as an Independent Consumer Representative for Cuisinart, Krups, LeCreuset, Rowenta, Braun and other high quality cookware and appliance manufacturers.

She has a massive collection of cookbooks, through which she constantly browses. Although she has pretty much given up on regularly watching most of the things on TV, she loves the cooking shows.

Throughout our life together, unless it was something from the outside grill, she cooked all of our meals, including appetizers, side dishes and desserts. However, long before her Alzheimer's diagnosis, I gradually began to take over the preparation of food.

At first, it was because she would simply forget to start dinner but then it was a matter of leaving out steps in the process or suddenly realizing that she didn't know what to do next. In addition, there was a safety factor when she would forget that something was cooking. This latter never caused anything more serious than having to discard a number of rather expensive pots and pans. Fortunately, many of them were gifts from manufacturers.

Eventually, I became the family chef. Having observed a master for all of those years, I had learned far more than I realized and I think I do a better than average good job.

At first, I tried to make at least the evening meal preparation a cooperative effort. I would decide on the entrée and buy it with the ingredients for a selection of accompaniments. I would assemble all the ingredients and then assign Mona responsibility for the simpler preparations, as well as I shamefully admit some things I just didn't want to do like cleaning up afterward.

Over time, two things happened. It became easier for me to do more and Mona lost interest in the process. She became content to set the table, wait to be served and to do the clean up. However, she didn't seem to realize that our roles had reversed.

If I commented that something I prepared tasted especially good, she would thank me for the compliment. Sometimes, she would ask if I liked something. When I said I did, she would tell me she fixed it especially for me. I would thank her. It was clear that she considered herself not only involved, but that I was merely a journeyman sous chef in her kitchen.

This is probably a good place to bring up another target of my vigilance, which may or may not be unique to Mona. I have jokingly referred to it as food vandalism. Vandalism is not really the correct term, since there is no malice or mischief involved. I don't think there is a word for inadvertent vandalism. However, it has many manifestations and the list is growing.

I am proud of my efficiency in shopping, especially my minimization of trips to the store and I try to buy fresh foods for a week at a time. I carefully check the "use by" dates on meat, poultry and seafood, and purchase them when I am sure that I will be able to use or freeze them well before they become questionable. However, that has required some modifications in conventional storage practices.

One day last summer I went to the store early in the morning and bought a roasting chicken and had it quartered, ground beef for burgers, large center cut pork chops, two brook trout, which I had filleted, and a two pound bag of frozen shrimp. When I came home, I put the shrimp and the chicken in the freezer and the rest in the refrigerator, planning on sautéing the trout for dinner.

Late that afternoon on a routine trip downstairs to check on Mona's status she proudly showed me what she had done to make my selection for dinner easier. All of my purchases were out of both the refrigerator and freezer, unwrapped and displayed the way entrees sometimes appear in refrigerated cases in restaurant dining rooms.

Mona arrayed the chops, trout and the defrosted chicken on plates and a platter, respectively. The ground beef was on a cutting board ready for forming into burgers and the entire two pounds of shrimp were in a large serving bowl of water, nearly thawed. It required prompt action to prevent the loss of at least six meals for two people.

I altered my storage facilities by buying two inexpensive Styrofoam coolers and several cooling packs, which you place in the freezer. When they are frozen, I put them in the coolers. I use the coolers for storage of no more than one day and change the freezer packs as needed. I put any frozen entrées in the large downstairs freezer, rather than the one in the refrigerator. This has probably nearly doubled my trips to the basement, but it works.

I try to avoid other instances of food vandalism by constant vigilance and that doesn't always work. Despite my efforts, Mona sometimes arbitrarily defrosts frozen vegetables, for which I have no immediate use. Fresh fruit and vegetables often mysteriously find their way into the freezer, and on occasion have made it to the microwave.

At least once, I placed a large salad without dressing in the refrigerator without dressing to remain crisp for dinner. When retrieved it for serving it was well dressed with cranberry soda, perhaps intended as faux vinaigrette.

Because Mona often wants to help in preparation, a related need for vigilance about which I have become fanatical, is the issue of sanitation. The most obvious is the problem of cross-contamination with chicken. It has reached the point where I never prepare a chicken dish in her presence.

That is not to say that Mona does not comprehend the concept of sanitation. In fact, she often seems obsessed by it. The problem is in the execution. She uses the nearest dish or utensil at hand, without regard to its inherent cleanliness or lack thereof. The real issue is that there is no way that I can watch her every move.

The result is that to be safe I must assume that all surfaces, dishes, glassware, pots and pans, service and tableware are contaminated. Therefore, I always wash everything before using. That includes washing an item I have just set down before using for a second time, unless I am the only person in the room.

Ironically, Mona is obsessed with cleaning up. If she spots serving dishes or preparation utensils in the sink, she will get up in the middle of the meal, go wipe them off (rather than wash them) and put them away dirty.

One must balance prevention, intervention and remedial strategies in order to maintain an acceptable level of stress and a semblance of normality. It is very important to realize that having no stress and complete normality is not achievable. One must go with the flow.

Keeping track of Mona's location during the day is not particularly difficult, since she is not a wanderer. It is really a matter of being alert to sounds.

When I hear the back door open and then don't hear anything else for several minutes, I look out my office window. If I don't see Mona, I go down to check. If I hear the front door open, I go to a front window to see where she is and I check on her every ten minutes. Mona has never gone more than a hundred yards from the front door.

If she wants to take a nap, I let her and I let her stay there until she wants to get up. If I see evidence that she has snacked extensively and she decides to go to bed for the night without dinner, I let her do that. Her weight has not varied more than two pounds between doctor's appointments in several years.

If I have to go out for a very brief time such as to the bank, post office or pharmacy and she wants to go with me, I take her. However if she wants to stay home, I let her but I always give her a note that says where I went and when I will be back.

If Mona has no appointments or other scheduled activities on Saturdays, she can sleep as late as she wants. Often if not usually, that is until afternoon. Sundays, she can sleep until eleven when she has to get up for Mass.

On those days, Mona always makes the bed and she is on her own to get dressed. Since she has no concept of what day it is, sometimes I have to suggest that she wear something else to go to church.

Once again, she is on her own those days although I try to spend most of Sunday with her.

Mona lives an apparently independent life, but she is always under supervision. Several medical professionals and social workers specializing in Alzheimer's care have questioned my approach. Some even suggest that it may not be appropriate. Nevertheless, when I point out that it works, they usually agree.

An increasing number of the medical professionals now believe that our approach to Mona's Alzheimer's Disease has maintained her functionality and that has significantly postponed her need for skilled care. I'd like to think she is *getting* skilled care, just from a different skill set.

At the same time, this approach interferes only minimally with my lifestyle. Although I would not do it in the evening, when Mona is sleeping in on Saturday or Sunday morning, I feel comfortable with leaving for a short while to go to the store. In fact, on a few occasions, I have scheduled a Saturday breakfast meeting. However, I always leave an explanatory note and return before eleven, which would be an early time for her to rise.

I understand that most people in the same situation as Mona and I are facing use a much different approach. They begin by restricting the Alzheimer's victim to a limited area of the house. They might use a room like our bedroom and add a few amenities like a reclining chair, but I feel that restricts and completely changes the nature of that familiar space.

Others might convert their living room into similar space, additionally altering the integrity of the home. I think that these courses of action would confuse, depress and perhaps even frighten the victim.

Many would place secure locks on exterior doors so that the victim could not get out, not because the victim is prone to wandering, but on the chance that some day they might just do that. I think that it is possible that some victims elect to wander because they feel imprisoned and challenged to express some level of independence.

Most Carekeepers who use the restriction approach add intensive monitoring and smothering vigilance, straining the psyche of both victim and Carekeeper until neither can bear the unrelieved pressure. Then, the only viable option is to trundle the victim off to a Nursing Home before he or she is ready to accept that, which imposes sufficient guilt on the Carekeeper to drive him or her to make long daily visits.

That scenario arrives soon enough. I think our approach is a sensible and more humane way to avoid that solution until it is clearly necessary.

Our approach is based on maintaining a lifestyle, gradually modifying things which are most essential and accommodating the rest. It is an effort to give Mona as much freedom to do what she wants to do, which is consistent with her health and safety. That means a very flexible, minimally structured schedule. It also means Mona's full access to every place in the house and yard as long as possible, as well as supervised access to places like Church, stores, theaters, restaurants and normal social activities.

So far it is working.

CHAPTER 6

▼

KNOW THE ENEMY

The fifth and final goal of our approach to Mona's care is to be even more aware of her physical and mental health than any one of her doctors, including a total awareness of all her medications. I intended to become the most knowledgeable person on such matters.

This includes staying as up to date as is practical on all Alzheimer's Disease information relevant to Mona, such as medications, treatments, research and related subjects. I intend to become as fully knowledgeable as possible on her medical issues. I also strive to engage in dialogue with the practitioners about both the physical and mental aspects of her condition. I think I can handle that.

I divided the information that I felt I needed to accumulate into the following classifications:

- General information regarding Alzheimer's Disease, including a working knowledge of applicable treatment, research and related subjects.

- Information about the monitoring and treatment of Mona's physical condition.

- Data from the clinical monitoring of the regression of Mona's mental condition with particular emphasis on her Alzheimer's Disease.

- My personal, 24/7/365, detailed observations of Mona's behavioral tendencies.

This task was far more difficult than I anticipated because of the inherently random nature of the disease. As I have discussed my experiences with others who have been close to an Alzheimer's victim, I have learned that we have had many of the same observations. Yet those with whom I have talked are usually struck as much as I by the very different things we have individually seen.

Not only do the symptoms of Alzheimer's appear in random order and frequency, but they also develop at different rates and reach different intensities. As a result, there is never any real sense of where the victim is in the course of the disease, despite the effort of some of the professionals to give the impression that there is. Their assessment is usually simplistic and vague, without even unanimity regarding the definition of terms. That makes planning very difficult.

For example, there is an evaluation tool used for determining the need of an Alzheimer's victim for Skilled Nursing Care, called a PRI. I will have more to say about this later. For the present, however, let me say that the Medical Community makes more of this than seems sensible at least to this Carekeeper.

First, although it consists of asking a set of very specific questions and recording the answers by checking the appropriate box, it requires specific training of a Registered Nurse to become an evaluator.

Secondly, since we all know there is no recovery from Alzheimer's, they require the administration of the test every three months even though the victim received the required score once. Of course, they charge a fee each time.

At a certain point, Mona exceeded the score indicating eligibility for Skilled Nursing Care. The next time she also met the criteria but with a lower score. The issue became which answers (which came from me) they would retroactively change to address the anomaly. I have no idea what they did because I refused to participate in such a travesty.

Nonetheless, given a different set of symptoms and their progression some of what you are reading in this book would not have been possible. For example if Mona had been a wanderer from the outset, this sort of physical environment would not have been possible. The same would have been true if she had been violent or if she had not retained her ability to feed herself and take care of the majority of her own personal needs.

Things would have also been much different if I had not been able to make major adjustments to my own lifestyle or still had to travel extensively or go to an outside office every day, as I did before Mona's diagnosis. Not all Carekeepers are able to have that much flexibility.

My effort to accumulate this knowledge base has been as comprehensive with regard to Mona's general health and as rigorous with regard to Alzheimer's Disease as practical without the tasks consuming me. After all, I am not personally in search of a cure or responsible for finding one.

That brings me to the first of my four classifications: the development of a personal understanding of the general information available on Alzheimer's Disease and the particular information regarding treatment, research and related subjects.

At this time, Alzheimer's has no cure. Some have asked me whether Alzheimer's is a new disease. Dr. Alois Alzheimer wrote so extensively on the disease more than one hundred years ago that in 1906 the illness was officially named Alzheimer's Disease. However, until people began living longer and the disease affected large numbers, science largely ignored the disease.

I believe that we ought to rid the world of all disease, but I think it should be noted that unless something is done soon, Alzheimer's would affect a larger segment of the population than HIV/Aids. Remember that Alzheimer's victims do not bring on their own illness. It is not behavior related like smoking, alcohol consumption, obesity or irresponsible sex. The Alzheimer's victim has no culpability for his or her condition and in fairness that should merit some consideration.

According to the press releases regarding significant breakthroughs in medications, they are the result of the expenditure of millions of dollars and dozens of years of Alzheimer's research. The reality is however, that they usually measure the efficacy of the few medicines introduced in terms of the number of months they will extend the victim's ability to go to the toilet unaided.

For the victim and those close to him or her, that is not very reassuring and certainly not a breakthrough. At the current rate, Alzheimer's victims will soon be able to go to the toilet unaided long past the point after which they are able to remember why they need to. That hardly seems like much progress over a period of more than one hundred years.

That which really surprised me was two-fold. First, an Internet search for "Alzheimer's Disease" using Google produced nearly three million references when I first tried in late 2002. That seemed an impossible assimilation task. Four years later, there were 7.3 million references. Second, I have been unable to find a single authoritative document that in layman's terms catalogues and summarizes the meaningful milestones in the search for either a means of diagnosis or a cure for this devastating illness. Unfortunately, that would be a very short document albeit quite useful.

That observation does not mean that there has been a lack of effort on the part of many heroic scientists. It does mean however, that until recent years the technology was not available to aid in the diagnosis or in the hypothesis for new treatments.

As a result, there is very little useful information for people like me, who believe that one can extend the quality of life for Alzheimer's victims by keeping them in a safe and comfortable home environment rather than rushing them to institutionalization. Unfortunately, that leaves the victims and their Carekeepers with "The Ultimate Do-It-Yourself Project".

The Alzheimer's Association does a great deal of very important work, but one must remember that developing "How To" manuals for Carekeepers is not one of their main priorities. They are properly, focused on raising independent funds for research, lobbying to raise sufficient awareness of the Disease to encourage government support for that research and directing those funds to the most promising areas. Everything else they do is fall-out.

In the period during which I have been more aware of their activities, there has also seemed to be an increased effort to provide formalized training for _professional_ caretakers. This is certainly a laudable objective and given the rapid increase in victims probably essential. However, the costs of taking _amateur_ Caretakers taking this training suggest that it may be just another aspect of their fundraising activities.

In saying that however, I realize that our approach is not always possible either because of the specific attributes of the victim's situation or the availability of a Carekeeper. However, one doesn't need a six-session course to do what we have done. That is the subject of this book.

Shortly after Mona's diagnosis, I attended two free public seminars for victims and caregivers, run by the local Alzheimer's Association. Although they had different names, they were pretty much the same and the emphasis seemed to be on either instilling fear concerning what could happen if the caregivers did not pay attention to the problem of wandering, or reducing guilt of the Carekeepers regarding the decision to institutionalize.

Although I was certainly not looking forward to that day, and knew that I would experience great sadness when it arrived I do not expect to have any guilt when it becomes necessary for Mona to move to a Skilled Nursing facility. I can say that because I intend to be certain that I have done the best job, of which I was capable for a long as possible.

I also intend to be sure that I make that decision on the basis that Mona needs something, which I cannot provide and not that it will make my life easier. I will say more about this in Chapter Eleven, which deals with that decision process.

I'd like to turn now to the classification of the on-going monitoring and treatment of Mona's physical condition. In many ways, this was the simplest of the four to master, perhaps because it proved to be quite interesting. My emphasis regarding Mona's physical health focused on avoiding her non-memory related disability and assuring that her death is not from some cause other than Alzheimer's Disease. The perverse or perhaps perverted irony of that is difficult to ignore.

I also try to monitor her struggle with depression, although I suspect that she ultimately will reach a point when she is no longer depressed. However, most of my attention goes toward finding indications useful in longer term planning. That is a large task.

The primary daily task of managing Mona's prescriptions and assuring that she takes them when she should is simple. However, I stay constantly on the alert for any news regarding each of her medications. For example, when stories first appeared regarding the ineffectiveness and actual danger of massive doses of Vitamin E and the problems with Bextra, Mona's doctor in whom I have complete trust, kidded me about noticing those issues before she did. I should point out that she has significantly more patients (bad pun) than I do.

I require that Mona's Primary Care Physician write any prescription recommended by other doctors. I make no decisions regarding non-prescription medicines without the concurrence of the PCP and assurance that she has added or removed them on her list of the things Mona is currently taking. In addition, I use just one pharmacy and check periodically to assure that their computers are up to date so that they will be able to detect dangerous interactions.

This does not seem like paranoia to me. I do the same with my own medications. It just makes sense.

Doctor's appointments are another common task. Obviously, I am responsible for transportation and even before Mona's diagnosis, I inserted myself into the appointment proper for several reasons. Mona cannot remember the questions to ask the doctor nor can she answer most of the questions the doctor asks. Worse yet, she cannot remember to tell me what the doctor said.

However, in my opinion, the most important benefit is that my presence and interaction with the doctor often stimulates conversation between us, which in turn often prompts the recollection of seemingly insignificant observations I may have made. This often proves be valuable.

In this way, I also carry information among the various medical professionals who see Mona. Once in awhile I am even able to point out something that one or more of the doctors didn't notice or recall. However, I often do not rely on my understanding of an issue and sometimes merely suggest phone consultations among them. Thus far, they have welcomed this approach.

A valuable side benefit of this approach has been that I have better insights regarding my own health and its care. The full burden for one's care should not be on the doctor. The patient should be a participant.

I do the same thing with all Mona's medical professionals, including her Psychiatrist, Gynecologist, Dermatologist, Podiatrist, Mammographer, Optometrist, Dentist and even Tipper's Veterinarian. They all appreciate my interest and my input. I was kidding about the Vet.

One small tip in this regard. Unless I absolutely cannot avoid it, I never accept any doctor's appointment other than his or her first of the day, even if that means Mona has to wait another week or two. I do that so that the doctor will not be behind schedule and feel rushed in treating Mona. I am so adamant on this that now the various secretaries automatically do that.

Now let us consider the medical evaluation of the most likely ultimate cause of Mona's death, her Alzheimer's. That is the task of a trained Clinical Psychiatrist, not a Primary Care Physician.

When the doctor diagnosed Mona with Alzheimer's he did not schedule a follow up visit. That did not mean that he would not see her again, only that it placed the burden of deciding when and how often to follow up on me.

It concerned me that I would lose intimate knowledge of Mona's condition that clinical monitoring provides. When I realized that, I immediately called to schedule an appointment. I may not be correct, but I had the impression that the doctor thought that was a bit unusual.

As I said earlier, I was concerned that since there is no cure and at least at that time, little in the way of medication and treatment after Mona's diagnosis the Psychiatric community might take an arm's length posture with her. After all, they might rightly assume that except for observation leading to diagnosis, they should spend their time on research. If that were the case, families and victims are on their own again participating in the "Ultimate Do-It-Yourself-Project".

Faced with that, I suspect that more families than should reach for the convenient answer of premature institutionalization. That decision, though expensive may become very attractive. New facilities, bright, cheery and with a full menu of activities are opening all the time. In some ways, I am sure that these places are often more attractive than the victim's home.

I will have much more to say on this subject in Chapter Eleven, but that is not what I think Mona wanted. I was determined to maintain the quality of her life in a comfortable and familiar setting for as long as possible. To do that safely, I needed all of the monitoring and feedback that I could obtain.

Perhaps my perception was not correct and because Mona's Primary Care Physician had made the earlier appointment as a consultation, the Psychiatrist assumed was that if the PCP felt it was necessary, she could ask for another consultation. In any event, I wanted Mona's Alzheimer's condition monitored by someone in the field, not her PCP. Fortunately, Mona's Primary Care Physician agreed with me.

At the follow up visit, I felt that the Psychiatrist was pleased at my interest and helpful in discussing possible treatment options. Two of those were new medications. The doctor had been involved in the development of both. The first, Aricept, was FDA approved and on the market.

The second was Mementine but now called Namenda, approved in Europe but not in the United States. To my surprise, the doctor openly discussed the option of getting the unapproved medication directly from Europe, despite the lack of US approval, and that it would cost $800 per month, via the apparently readily available international black market. The only problem was that the FDA had not yet accepted its actual benefit and since it was unapproved, none of the available prescription drug programs would pay for it.

We decided to begin the Aricept at once and wait until the FDA approved Mementine. Then when it became domestically available, her drug plan covered it. I was comfortable with that because the two drugs worked together, rather than as alternatives.

With many drugs like Aricept, the patient begins the medication slowly, with the dosage increased over time until it reaches the desired level with the progress monitored. Mona began the Aricept with a dosage of 5 mg for three or four weeks, which she tolerated well.

During the afternoon of the day that we increased the dosage to 10 mg, Mona became very anxious and I urged her to go to bed. Later that night while I was asleep, she arose and went downstairs. The lights were out. As she tried to return upstairs in the dark and tripped on the bottom step and fell, striking her head, producing a very small cut, but a great deal of blood. That was unsettling for both of us.

The next day her Primary Care Physician took Mona off the Aricept. About two months later it was restarted at the 5 mg level and has remained at that level ever since without incident. We are now considering an increase in the dosage.

During the same appointment in which we discussed the two medications, the Psychiatrist posed another possibility. He was involved in a number of clinical trials of potential Alzheimer's treatments. He thought that Mona might qualify for one of several upcoming trials.

Although I understood that the medications studied were unproven to help, that half of the participants received a placebo rather than the medicine and that Mona's participation in the study required considerable demands on me, I was eager to pursue this option. There was a modicum of altruism in that feeling, regarding a contribution to research to benefit others in the future, but my main motivation was admittedly selfish.

That was due to my prior feeling that there was a tendency among doctors involved in Alzheimer's to abandon the victims once they made the diagnosis even if that diagnosis is the non-diagnosis of "inconclusive". I say that not totally as criticism, since in some ways it is understandable.

They can prescribe drugs like Aricept, but those drugs can only extend the decline in the victim's condition, not improve it and those medications are most effective when the regimen is started early rather than at the stage which Mona had already reached. There is no memory therapy to apply and no recovery. It must be easy for them to rationalize that the vast majority of their time should be devoted to research where perhaps they can make a difference.

Can I understand that? Yes. Is it helpful to the Carekeeper? No.

I saw the clinical trials with the inherently forced monitoring of Mona as a way for me to avoid that abandonment. As soon as I realized that I began to push very hard to have Mona included in any clinical study that was appropriate and for which she qualified. After six months of nagging by me, Mona entered a clinical study starting November 2003, just under one year after her diagnosis.

The study was a trial for a drug called Valproate to determine whether in certain dosages it would help Alzheimer's victims. Valproate has been around for over forty years as a treatment for seizures so its inherent safety did not seem to be an issue.

Even though I knew that Mona had only a 50% chance of getting the Valproate and not a placebo, she could continue to take the Aricept concurrently. That made the approach more attractive.

However, as I said, for me the most important benefit of the Valproate trial was the clinical monitoring of Mona for the two to three years of the trial and that I would have access to the feedback from that monitoring. That eliminated one of my biggest fears.

Since it is unlikely that Alzheimer's victims would even remember they were in a study, one might ask why it is necessary to give anyone a placebo. The answer is that to be in the study Mona had to have a study partner who could provide the information and respond to the questions of the study administrators. That would be me and they didn't want me to know whether she was getting the medicine or the placebo.

However, there were some initial hurdles to clear.

One of the standard tests given to Alzheimer's victims is the Mini Mental Status Exam (MMSE). It consists of a number of questions. A perfect score on the test would be thirty points. Before Mona entered the study, her score was twelve, the minimum allowed.

However, at Mona's first study appointment she went off with a nurse for testing. While I was talking to the doctor in charge of the actual study, the nurse came in and said, somewhat cryptically, "I was only able to get eleven".

The doctor thought for a minute and replied, "Make it twelve". I am sure he thought I had not understood the conversation and he did not explain. We cleared the first hurdle. The second was more difficult.

As with the Aricept, they introduced Valproate (or the placebo) gradually, taking several weeks to reach full dosage. When she went to the third level, she had a strong reaction, becoming very agitated and anxious. I called her PCP immediately. Mona was obviously on the Valproate and not the placebo. Her doctor took her off it.

At first, the study people were upset with this turn of events and they were considering taking Mona out of the study. Fortunately, they found some others around the country that had also been unable to tolerate the medicine and none was taking the placebo. They decided to create a third study group of those not on anything.

Although I didn't know it beforehand, I soon learned that the task of the study partner is far more onerous than that of the participant. Mona and I were in the study for two years. They monitored her progress, or more realistically, her decline in several ways. At six-month intervals, they administered a battery of tests to Mona, which I will discuss later. During the first of these sessions I met with the Psychiatrist who was in charge of the trial on general issues and then with a Nurse who asked a number of questions about my perceptions of Mona and my reactions to them.

There also were interim sessions halfway between the extensive tests for Mona during which they checked her general physical condition. However, these sessions were much more demanding on me.

Each time, the Senior Nurse asked me more than a hundred detailed questions about Mona's behavior designed to track trends in the intensity and frequency of the behavior and the effect of that behavior on me. She asked if I had observed a certain behavior. If I answered yes, I had five choices about frequency and five about my reaction.

She entered this information carefully forms for evaluation later. I once asked if the purpose of the study was to get me to answer each with "Yes", "Constantly" and "It drives me crazy." The nurse said she didn't think so.

That was both tedious and interesting. When we finished the questions, a second interviewer concentrated more on the way I was thinking about and dealing with the situation. In typical fashion for such people, she never told me how <u>she</u> thought I was dealing with it. That would have been very helpful.

Starting with the session including Mona's second battery of tests, the Senior Nurse asked me a smaller subset of the more comprehensive list of questions and there was a shorter interview with the second nurse conducting a shorter interview.

Finally, the Senior Nurse called me every six weeks with eight to ten different questions. The process was fascinating.

I received the results of Mona's testing every six months. The following is a history of those testing sessions:

> They did two kinds of testing. The first was the Mini Mental Status Exam (MMSE). It consisted of a number of questions. A perfect score on the test would be thirty points. Mona's results were:

November 2003	12
May 2004	11
November 2004	8
May 2005	5
November 2005	1

The second test consisted of five categories, generally making up what I understood to constitute Executive Function. Each was measured on a scale of six levels: No Impairment, Very Mild, Mild, Moderate, Moderately Severe, and Severe. Since these were subjective judgments, they were not precise. An appearance of improvement indicates that imprecision, not improvement. There was no summary evaluation. These were the categories and scores:

Remembering Written Instructions

November 2003	Severe
May 2004	Severe
November 2004	Severe
May 2005	Severe
November 2005	Severe

Comprehension of Speech

November 2003	Mild
May 2004	Moderate
November 2004	Moderate
May 2005	Moderately Severe
November 2005	Moderately Severe

Word Finding Difficulty

November 2003	Mild
May 2004	Moderately Severe
November 2004	Moderate
May 2005	Moderately Severe
November 2005	Moderately Severe

Language Use

November 2003	Mild
May 2004	None
November 2004	None
May 2005	Moderately Severe
November 2005	Moderately Severe

Executive Function (This is not what I have described earlier as Executive Function, but a simple maze through which a line must be drawn without touching a wall or lifting the pencil. Errors are counted).

November 2003	None
May 2004	None
November 2004	None
May 2005	One
November 2005	Two

Following the November 2004 testing, which represented a year in the study, the Senior Nurse told me that the team would review Mona's case for one of three possible outcomes:

- Continuation of her participation in the study.

- Removal of her from the study.

- Move of her into a different study.

She also told me that I should expect the decision within a few weeks. However, when I didn't hear anything for over a month, I called and arranged an interview with Dr. Tariot, who made the initial diagnosis and was the head of the department and the study. Early in that interview, he gave Mona an MMSE test on which she scored five, a decline of 38% in two months. I suspected that meant she would not be eligible for a different study. It turned out that my suspicion was correct.

The conversation was a strange one. The doctor began by saying that he knew my participation in the study was onerous and that he appreciated my willingness to do it. I figured he was leading up to telling me that he dropped Mona from the study, which was the last thing I wanted to happen.

I decided my best strategy was to agree with him, but to make the case that despite the burden I thought I had something to contribute and was willing to let Mona continue. I also stressed how valuable the feedback from the study was in helping me to care for Mona.

After about five minutes of this, we realized we both wanted the same thing. Apparently, my performance in terms of dedication and insight was somewhat above the norm. The bottom line was that Mona would stay in the study to its end. I needed to figure out how to continue to get feedback after that happened, but I had some time.

The doctor made an additional recommendation during that appointment. He suggested that we start Mona on Namenda, the drug that was previously unapproved and available only from Europe. She began that treatment with no complications of intolerance for the drug. However, I saw no difference in her condition.

As might be expected, the richest source of unevaluated data on Mona's struggle with Alzheimer's is my personal, full time observation of her under all conditions. The anomaly that during the search for a diagnosis doctors routinely ignored it was not lost on me.

Recalling and recounting those observations is often depressing and frustrating. However, our participation in the study provided the necessary discipline for me to mine that treasure of information and have it refined by professionals.

On an ongoing basis, I have tried very hard to record and catalog my personal, 24/7/365, detailed observations of Mona's behavioral tendencies. There were three principal purposes for this.

I believed the first was to keep our children and extended family informed of all aspects of Mona's illness. I considered that the second was for my analysis in order to develop coping strategies for them. Finally, I thought the third was to develop intelligence and present it to the medical people so they had an idea of the progression of the disease and Mona's concomitant regression as a person.

Both recording and cataloging are more difficult and time consuming than they might seem. The data is by definition anecdotal and when looked at as individual instances, often trivial. From the perspective of the Carekeeper, a day's worth of trivia loses its triviality. That phenomenon is difficult to explain and even harder to defend.

My problem was a difficulty in evaluating the data for its significance. Frankly, at first I was collecting too much data that was not. When I discovered that, I went the other way ignoring and tolerating many things, which were actually artifacts of the disease.

Along with that came a perceived difficulty in communicating with the children and their spouses. I began to feel that they interpreted my recitation of instances of Mona's behavior as tattling and even disloyalty on my part to Mona. They wanted facts, not anecdotes, and I began to feel that I was indeed becoming a whiner. In effect, *my* behavior was becoming more counter-productive. That wasn't helping anyone.

My efforts to record and catalog my personal, detailed observations of Mona's behavioral tendencies were very appropriate. The purposes for my doing it were mostly wrong and I needed to fix that.

The proper and exclusive purpose for that activity is to do the analysis necessary to develop coping strategies for them, and that is an on-going process. In fact, when my analysis no longer results in rational and effective coping strategies, I must turn the job over to someone else.

Reporting those strategies, rather than the raw data to both the family and the medical professionals is more valid and tangible enough for them to grasp and perhaps offer suggestions for modification.

Changes in behavior are frustratingly random and difficult to evaluate. Some things, which appear to be significant, prove to be merely anomalies. The reverse is also true.

Sometimes it seems impossible to design a coping strategy for something. Then when I finally do come up with one, the behavior has disappeared. With experience, one finds that on occasion the best coping strategy is simply to ignore the behavior.

I will cover this subject in more detail in the next chapter.

CHAPTER 7

▼

SYMPTOMS, SYMPTOMATIC BEHAVIORS AND BEHAVIORS

I am among those who lament the loss of precision with the English language. It is exceedingly rich with a vocabulary several times the size of any other. Despite that wealth of choice, or perhaps because of it people constantly confuse one another by failing to select the precise word. I often try to do my little bit to clarify such things.

Webster defines symptom as "a condition in the body or in its behavior, noted by the patient, suggesting the presence of injury or disease". One can clinically measure conditions in this context, like temperature and blood pressure. Behaviors are obviously immeasurable observations. This symptomatology is part of the diagnostic process and I refer to those phenomena as "Symptomatic Conditions" and "Symptomatic Behaviors".

Once there is a diagnosis, most of such conditions and behaviors are determined to be resultant, rather than symptomatic. I make this distinction for the same reason I made one between patient and victim earlier in the book. For me a patient is one undergoing treatment for a cure. His or her symptoms are clues that may prove to be nothing. Victims, their conditions and their behaviors are stark realities.

We are well beyond symptomatology and its implied speculation here. This is day-to-day dealing with the practical details of Carekeeping. These are lifestyle changes and much more than that. They require re-thinking long held assumptions and beliefs. They require adapting to the obvious and sometimes not so obvious conclusions they force.

There is a great deal more to Dementia than forgetting people's names.

Of course, I had known some people with Dementia; my paternal grandfather for one, but that was over sixty years ago when I was fourteen or so. My grandfather was seventy-five when he died, my age when I began this book and ancient by the standards of that period.

My mother had some form of Dementia when in her mid-nineties, but it was complicated by years of severe clinical depression following my father's death. One might argue logically and convincingly that she just didn't care enough any more to exert the effort to remember things.

I have had friends whose husbands or wives suffered from Dementia and I have noticed that often those victims in effect became invisible. Their friends had no sense of the progression, or more accurately perhaps, retrogression of the Disease. The result is that they make assumptions. Most of those assumptions are incorrect, which the Carekeepers involved had to learn by themselves.

Now Mona and I were the ones in danger of becoming invisible. The primary purpose of this book is to help Carekeepers as they deal with the "Ultimate Do-It-Yourself Project".

My general assumption about Alzheimer's was that its progression would be rather orderly and linear and that specific behaviors would begin all at once and in some logical sequence. Instead, those behaviors develop at different rates, randomly, with no schedule, sequence or pattern.

In the first few months after Mona's diagnosis, I realized that although these assumptions were not totally right, they were not very wrong either. More important was the realization that there are a great many more factors to consider and learn.

In addition, with more than a modicum of arrogance I thought I could deal with all those situations in the same way I have dealt with other problems over the years. That is, by acknowledging them, defining them, planning a remedy and executing it. To some degree that was correct because I was realistic and accepted whatever help there might be.

I also trusted my instincts, once I accumulated all the facts I could. However, there was a great deal to learn and I want to make it clear that the analysis which follows was made the hard way, by living it and not something I figured out at the outset.

My first major discovery was that the analogy that dealing with an Alzheimer's victim is similar to dealing with a young child is fundamentally incorrect.

This information is particularly important to the Carekeeper, from the standpoint of both the victim's safety and the mental health of the Carekeeper. Within it also lies the secret of making this arrangement work.

One of the most fundamental, inherent attributes of human beings is that we are all teachers. We have a strong internal drive to share what we know both in the abstract and the specific and to communicate that to others who have not yet learned it.

We also incorrectly congratulate ourselves on the efficacy of our teaching in developing the skills and knowledge of others. While that is no doubt partially true, the overwhelming reason for any success in teaching lies in the ability or desire of the student to learn.

Learning is dependent on memory. It is a cumulative process and the information collected is interconnected, associative and supplemental. While the child's memory is expanding at an astounding rate, the memory of the Alzheimer's victim is rapidly diminishing, with those connections, associations and supplements being lost. Soon their ability to learn is lost or from our perspective, they become unteachable. One must accept that reality.

When I said that my assumption was that the progression of the disease would be orderly, I meant that I thought I would see a steady and somewhat logical increase in the number of things that Mona would not be able to remember. That was indeed the case. However, there was no apparent logic involved in chronology, importance or subject matter for the loss. In addition, I did not realize the number of ways Dementia would affect so many other aspects of her life.

When I said that my expectation was that specific problems would arrive all at once I meant traumatic things like a sudden inability for her to dress herself, bathe, drive, go outside alone, or feed herself. Those things all occur in the progression of the disease, but sometimes you think you see them and you really don't. The greater surprises were that there were many other things to think about and some of the ways to deal with them were far different than they appeared.

Is all of this scary? You're damned right!

I think that it is useful to classify the various behaviors, which I have observed in Mona as well as some that I haven't. That will help me to present a more coherent picture of the progression of the disease. It may also help the reader to understand what is related and what is not.

However before I begin, I must make something abundantly clear. Eventually with Alzheimer's virtually all behavior by the victim will become unacceptable, either inherently or because of the danger it presents to the victim or others including of course the Carekeeper.

That is just the way it is and the Carekeeper must accept that reality. No amount of patience, scolding or coping will change or even delay that reality. Deal with that, but deal with it in a kind and loving way by merely accepting responsibility for the task and moving on.

A good example of this is the matter of driving. At the point when you realize that isn't a good idea, quietly do something about it. If he or she got lost, don't say, "Well, that the last time that will happen!" The experience no doubt terrified him or her and they don't need to be hurt as well.

When you have the opportunity, quietly take the keys. Put them away in a secure place and with no further mention of it assume the task of chauffeur. That was the only possible solution anyway, so don't make a big deal about it.

I will discuss Mona's case in the context of the following classifications of Alzheimer's Disease behaviors:

- Behaviors that are strictly memory related.

- Behaviors related to the struggle to cope with impaired memory.

- Behaviors that are related more to loss of Executive Function than memory.

- Behaviors not directly related to impaired memory or Executive Function.

- Behaviors common to Alzheimer's Disease not yet exhibited by Mona.

Within each classification, I will mention how I have tried to help her, some of which worked as well as some that didn't. Some are things I am doing to help myself. Many things I will say may be obvious, but some will not.

I have come to realize that although some behaviors beget behaviors they all don't and that is quite revealing. Mona always had a great many friends. In terms of those I would describe as close friends, she had far more than I did and she was always very generous of her time with them. If they were ill, she visited them often taking an entire meal that she had prepared. When they needed transportation, she was a willing chauffer. Moreover, when she knew they were alone she would always call to cheer them up.

When Mona first began to demonstrate discernible Dementia and especially after her diagnosis, I assumed these people would want to know. I called those who I knew were particularly close and when I ran into others, I would bring them up to date. They all thanked me for calling but not one has ever called or mentioned it when we have met them on some occasion. I find that very strange and more than a little sad. They have lost a great deal.

Allow me to tell you again a bit about their loss by saying that Mona is a college graduate, with some advanced degree study, who taught high school English and Social Studies. She has been an excellent wife and mother. She was active in the Girl Scouts and was President of the Women's Guild at our church.

She was a self-taught, accomplished chef, and when Cuisinart Food Processors came on the market, the company recruited her as a trainer, demonstrator and instructor. She read extensively and kept current with world and national affairs. She was a skilled event planner and a highly competent event manager, with an excellent memory for detail. She also has proven to be a good actress, particularly when she is not on any stage.

Behaviors, which are strictly memory related

This classification is imprecise and needs further clarification. Memory affects nearly everything we do. I do mean the loss of specific memories of people and relationships, events and their significance, places and their relative locations. I also mean the loss of long held attitudes, preferences and habits. Moreover, I also mean the role of memory in connection with one's self-protection and other sensory functions.

The obvious things lost are names, events and places. The less obvious are vocabulary, pronunciation and definitions of words used without the assistance of a clear context. However, for Alzheimer's victims that eventually means not being able to remember the words at the beginning of a sentence until they reach the end. Therefore, they don't understand what someone is telling them or even what they are saying themselves.

Mona lost memories of events first, perhaps because it was difficult to fake their details. She did better with people, although I quickly realized her strategy. She could recognize them as people she knew, but often wasn't able to come up with a name or a context. To finesse that and head off questions for which she didn't have answers, Mona would try to pre-empt the conversation by quickly asking them about their children often out of necessity without using their names.

Gradually, that ability eroded and Mona replaced it with a strategy once again of taking the offensive with an effusive greeting accompanied by hugs. This was obviously disconcerting to her friends when she repeated the same greeting ten minutes later.

Before long, Mona had trouble remembering the status of family members who she didn't see often. She couldn't remember that people had died, like her mother or father and my father, mother or sister.

This is frustrating for Mona, and for me it is the loss of a conversation partner and the sharing of nearly sixty years of joint memories. Mona now lives exclusively in the present.

The identities of our children and grandchildren confuse her and although she knows that I am very close to her, she isn't always sure of what our relationship is or where I live. Ironically, that does not result in her being defensive or mistrustful of them or me.

Mona began to lose not just thoughts, but vocabulary. The vocabulary loss became noticeable as it affected syntax, particularly in the use of opposite gender names and or personal pronouns. She began to refer to herself in the third person. Then there were episodes of incoherent or unintelligible statements or questions. Now there is often just gibberish.

Mona's verbal skills began to deteriorate around the time of her diagnosis, although much earlier she exhibited lapses into confabulation, which is another by-product of memory loss. Initially, it was an attempt to mask memory loss by inserting statements, which fit the context but are simply untrue.

I became aware of this phenomenon when Mona was in the hospital for her alcohol problems. She would begin to tell something, forget what it was and "confabulate". That is to say, she would make something up occasionally related in some way, but often out of whole cloth.

Confabulation is a defense mechanism and in the early stages, she did it logically so that what she said <u>sounded</u> all right. If one didn't know the facts, it was believable. Over time, the ability to reach for something logical deteriorates and the result becomes obviously incorrect. Later it results in pseudo sentences, with inflection and emphasis, which are essentially gibberish.

Although Mona doesn't show it outwardly, I believe that this is very frustrating and upsetting to her. She will often start to say something and after some difficulty will just say, "Never mind … I don't know what I am talking about". I don't think she means that in the usual sense.

Recently, another version of this has emerged. When there are only the two of us present, Mona will suddenly ask me something like, "What does she need to do with that?" I have learned that usually "she" is a reference to herself, but I still need more information so I ask, "With what?" She sometimes responds indignantly with, "I don't know". I haven't been able to handle that one adequately and often I feel trapped in an endless Abbott and Costello routine.

At first, I tried to address these problems as a game of Charades looking for clues and suggesting answers. Sometimes that was effective, but the success was short lived because her prior thought and connection had been lost.

Mona has begun to withdraw from conversational situations even with me, making an excuse that she does not feel well or is tired and is going to bed. If I go upstairs later, as often as not the light is on in the bedroom and she is up sometimes watching TV but often just puttering.

During the day, she sometimes attempts to read the newspaper and some magazines although I am not sure that she is still able. The TV is usually on, although I don't think she really pays any attention to it. She cannot distinguish programs from commercials and several times, I have seen her watching foreign language broadcasts that I know she does not understand.

I also noticed two new behaviors, which strike me as interesting. I don't know if they are related, but they began about the same time. I think that they apparently resulted from the loss of some level of inhibition in Mona's thought or memory process.

I have known Mona since 1948 and one of the first things she told me was that she never had dreams. She said that as a child she often had disturbing nightmares and had prayed that she wouldn't dream. She said the prayers had worked. However, since I knew that everyone has dreams, I assumed she had just conditioned herself to forget her dreams when she awoke.

Then one night after her diagnosis, Mona had the first nightmare I ever recall her having, although she was not clear as to its content. Since then this has happened every week or two. She becomes frightened, calls out, but quickly recovers and goes back to sleep.

The second observation is even more interesting to me. In the nearly fifty-five years that we have been married, I have never known Mona to talk in her sleep. Now she does it quite often.

As I have said when awake, Mona's verbal skills have deteriorated so that she is generally unintelligible, sometimes just confusing words and sometimes speaking in gibberish. However, when she talks in her sleep, she is lucid, completely coherent and the "conversations" last several minutes. She and I even have a dialogue sometimes.

Obviously, I am only hearing one side of the conversation but as when one overhears a phone call there is a perceived continuity. A few times, she has said something funny and laughed.

I shared these observations with the doctor in charge of the Alzheimer's Unit at Strong Hospital. I also told the doctor who conducted the medication clinical trials that included Mona. Each expressed only polite interest. I sometimes think that research people are only interested in their own observations. They can miss a lot that way.

Memory also protects us. It allows us to walk around our homes in the dark without a care, find a tiny keyhole with a key at night and do a myriad of other things without danger. We have a chair with wide wooden arms in our family room in which Mona has been sitting for years. One day she sat down in the chair and hit her "funny bone" on the arm. A little while later, she stood up to get something. When she sat down again, she whacked her elbow a second time.

That little vignette demonstrated something that I had never considered before. A person without Dementia, who strikes his or her elbow on the arm of a chair, is without realizing it thereafter protected from doing it again by memory. Eventually, that loss of protection extends to things that are too hot or sharp. For an Alzheimer's victim that may amount to a loss of any rational fear. Alzheimer's victims don't have that protection.

This non-verbal aspect of memory loss is the way it affects our every day living. We process many odors, temperature changes, peripheral vision images and a seemingly infinite variety of sounds, some of which we have never heard before. Memory is essential for a great many more important things than recalling what one had for lunch.

That reminds me of another aspect of Mona's memory loss, which has to do with food. She has forgotten that she doesn't like some foods that I like. In a perverse way, this is something that has made my life easier.

Although rhubarb was the only thing that Mona would *never* eat, she did have distinct preferences and some of them were in conflict with mine. One day I decided to test Mona's memory of food preferences.

Although I preferred large sea scallops, she liked the smaller bay scallops. However, neither of us really disliked the alternatives. However, she usually bought and prepared the smaller ones. Sort of a "ties you lose" proposition.

Without mentioning it, I bought and prepared sea scallops and served them one evening in linguine nests. My first test was a rousing success. We never had bay scallops again.

The same was true of a number of foods with which we had different preferences. Now I can drink buttermilk whenever I like, have lima beans on occasion and I don't have to eat peppers, broccoli or cauliflower. There hasn't been an onion in our house in years.

I can fix tubular pasta because she has forgotten that she thinks it tastes funny and she now loves sour cream on her baked potato. Why this has happened baffles me.

Another manifestation of memory loss leading to different behaviors has to do with forgetting the primary purpose of something. This extends to some things that are basic elements of every day life.

The last paragraph introduces what has become Mona's signature behavior, which has become an obsession.

Over some period of time, Mona had succeeded in putting away all of the everyday cloth table napkins in places where they could not be found without several people spending a day or two turning the house upside down. Prior to that, she had done the same thing with all the dishtowels and I had begun to use paper towels exclusively.

Unable to find any napkins one day Mona began to substitute paper towels folded once, straight down the middle. At first that seemed like a reasonable strategy and not anything that offended me.

Before long, she began to use the paper towels, now folded twice to form a square a quarter of the size of a full towel, as coasters. Then things got out of hand. Soon every dish, figurine, lamp and plant had a paper towel coaster under it.

I would go to the cupboard to get a plate and discover a folded paper towel under each plate in every stack. I began to hide the paper towels I bought in the trunk of the car, waiting until Mona was distracted to retrieve them one roll at a time, which I would place just out of her sight on top of the refrigerator.

Like many people, Mona always used Kleenex or some similar product. I probably need not point out that doing that is an expensive way to buy essentially the same product found in roll form. So when Mona began spending part of her waking hours cutting the sheets of Kleenex into squares, stacking them and using them far a wide range of purposes, I changed the form in which I bought Kleenex.

I had to stop buying Kleenex because Mona immediately processed it into useless square half sheets. She had forgotten the primary purpose of the Kleenex as well as the paper towels.

Undaunted, she shifted her raw material to the toilet tissue, quickly converting roll after roll into neat little stacks of individual sheets. That led her to a second step in processing the paper towels. Instead of folding them into quarters, she began to cut them.

Every drawer, cupboard, table and counter in the house had stacks of paper towels cut in quarters or toilet tissue sheets detached from their rolls. When Mona became bored, she just added to her inventory.

Paper products were becoming a major item in our operating budget. I started to buy cheaper towels in larger packages to control the cost. Eventually, I began to buy the least expensive paper towels that I could find. However, I admit that I didn't go that far with toilet tissue, although I did begin to buy two grades. You know, one for show and one for whatever.

This particular behavior is not however, limited to Mona.

Last summer a friend of ours died and we went to the wake in Syracuse. He was a very popular Judge with legions of friends and passing through the line to greet his widow took a couple of hours. When it began to rain, they brought as many as they could inside the Funeral Home doubling the lines back on one another several times.

A college friend of mine was quite a bit behind us in the line but in the cramped quarters, we kept passing each other. Although I hadn't seen him for many years, I knew that his wife had Alzheimer's Disease. Each time we passed, we would talk a little about it.

Mona was getting tired so I had her sit down in a chair where I could keep an eye on her as I wended my way. One time when I passed Paul, he was laughing. He pointed at Mona and said, "My wife does that all the time. Day and night. Week after week".

On the table next to Mona was a large box of Kleenex and one at a time, she was carefully tearing each sheet it half.

Another example of forgetting the purpose of things had to do with Cranberry Soda, which became Mona's beverage of choice and much more. She has used it as a marinade, a salad dressing, an ice cream topping, a dish detergent and many applications that are more creative.

I think there is another aspect of this sort of thing that is really more of a philosophy than a behavior. Mona came to believe in "everything in something else's place". I will let your imagination deal with that and you may feel content in thinking that whatever you imagine probably has happened.

At one point, our microwave stopped working. I am sure that Mona put something in it that she shouldn't have and shorted it. Since it was larger than we really needed and a built in unit that also included the venting system for the stove and its light, I decided to leave it in place and functionally replace it with a smaller, counter mounted model. The real logic of that decision had to do with the fact that I knew I would be moving when Mona ultimately entered a care facility.

Mona never figured out that the old microwave didn't work. I would often find things in it that she had obviously tried to microwave. Sometimes the timer would be running down from its maximum of ninety-nine minutes. Sometimes I would find the day's newspaper in there, probably because it was wet when she brought it in and she was trying to dry it.

Our daughter Maryellen once said that Mona had at least one of every kitchen gadget. That may be an exaggeration, but often I would pick up one of them, the purpose of which I could not determine and ask her what it was. In most cases, she had forgotten.

One of her best gadgets was a special ice cream scoop. It had a hollow handle filled with a liquid, which could retain heat. The idea was that you would run hot water over the handle and it would be easy to scoop the hardest ice cream. Inexplicably, Mona suddenly began to keep putting the scoop in the freezer.

Here is another, perhaps more dramatic example of forgetting the purpose of something.

Sunday Mass has always been a major part of Mona's life. Very early in the regression of Alzheimer's Mona lost the ability to keep track of what day it was. She would try to look at the newspaper for the answer, but that is circular logic and begs the question, "Is this today's paper?" The importance of Mass to her was made evident in her question every day, "Have we been to Mass yet?"

Mona liked the crowds at Mass and especially the children, but soon the reason why she was there began to elude her. She could not follow the readings in the Missal or the sense of Homily. She did however find things to keep her attention.

She took notice of everyone she could within view and when she saw someone she thought she knew, she asked who it was. Since I didn't know all of the people she knew, sometimes I couldn't help her and she found that very annoying. She eventually became rather critical of people, particularly if they were overweight or obviously colored their hair. Unfortunately, at about the same time she apparently forgot how to whisper.

Mona also could be both helpful and flattering. Alzheimer's had liberated her of many inhibitions and even at important points of the service; she might tuck in an exposed label or adjust the jacket for a person sitting nearby. On occasion, she might tap a stranger on the shoulder to tell her that she liked her dress.

One day when we arrived and were seated, she said excitedly, "Look who is there!" and pointed to the front of the church. I finally figured out that she thought a member of the choir was her sister Mary Gene. I could see a vague resemblance although the woman in question was about forty years younger and Mary Gene lives ninety miles away.

Mona adamantly refused to accept that it wasn't Mary Gene and all through Mass, whenever the woman looked her way, Mona waved. That routine has gone on for about four years. It reached the point that the woman actually seemed to be looking for Mona, although it may have been one of those cases where no matter how many times you tell yourself not to look at something, you can't resist and look anyway. At least the woman has not waved back. Yet.

Eventually, even receiving Communion became confusing for Mona. Nowadays, most people exercise the option of taking the host from the Eucharistic Minister in their hands and placing it in their own mouths. They then move to the Minister with the chalice and take a sip of wine from it. Some do a variation on that of that, taking the host and dipping it into the chalice.

At first, Mona became uncertain of what to do with the host when she had it in her hand. She would look to me for help. I would demonstrate and she would follow. Occasionally however, I would find that when we returned to our seats Mona still had the host in her hand. I would gently advise her as to what to do and she was fine.

One morning, Mona took the host and noticed that person ahead of her had dipped hers in the chalice so Mona followed suit. When I got to the woman with the chalice, her eyes were like saucers and there was panic on her face.

As I took the chalice, I saw the problem. Mona had not dipped the host into the chalice; she had deposited it there and gone on. Perhaps with Divine Guidance, I calmly took a large gulp of wine, which included Mona's host. As I handed back the chalice, the woman looked in and sighed a fervent "Thank you".

Over time, Mona seemed to have a less of a compulsive attitude about attending Mass. Whether it had become more difficult to be in crowds, or the ritual became more confusing, I don't know.

In any case, it became more difficult to get her up to go. While "we have to go to Mass" had been the easiest way to get her out of bed, she began to respond with "just let me sleep a little longer" or "I don't feel well" to "I don't want to go". She usually responded eventually, but sometimes I just couldn't get her to go and went on alone.

That didn't bother me too much. Somehow, I think God probably cuts Alzheimer's victims a little slack even at Sunday Mass. In some ways, it was a reminder to me that the person who looked like Mona was no longer she.

There is no pattern in things Mona forgets. The same is true for those she does not. Of course, there are more of the former than the latter but here are some examples.

As I mentioned earlier, Mona no longer grasps the concept of Instant Replay on TV. She loves watching golf and football, but when they replay a long putt or a long run, she shouts advice and encouragement at the runner or the ball each time.

On the other hand, when Tipper escapes from the confines of our backyard because Mona has left the gate open and tantalizes us with the threat that she is running away, Mona remembers that Tipper always heads west up the street and ends up in the backyard of the third house on the left. She grabs the leash and returns quickly with the docile, but exhilarated dog by her side.

I prefer to read the daily paper while relaxing before dinner at the end of the day. Because Mona began to put the day's paper out with the trash, my only defense has been to grab it first thing in the morning and hide it in my office until I go back downstairs at the end of the day.

I guess I can understand this one because Mona reads the same books and magazines day after day without ever finishing them.

Conversely, whenever Mona gets into car she immediately looks in the glove box to see if she has left any breath mints there as she used to do.

These are some of the thousands of reasons that make Alzheimer's such a confounding and exasperating disease.

Behaviors which are related to the struggle to cope with impaired memory

When Mona returned from rehab at Conifer Park in early 1994, long before her Alzheimer's diagnosis, she was suffering short-term memory problems. Many medical appointments and therapy sessions were part of her treatment, and she had to attend the ninety mandatory AA meetings in ninety days.

Mona was a little paranoid that she would do or not do something that might result in a return to Conifer Park, so to help her keep things straight I bought her one of those Week-At-A-Glance Calendar desk books. Mona really appreciated that. It is not clear when that simple aid became an obsession, but it definitely did.

The first expansion of the concept was Mona's perceived need for a purse-sized version of the desk book. That seemed reasonable. Then Mona started to accumulate calendars, most of them the 8 x 12, or 10 x 15 sizes, on the theory that there should be one downstairs and one upstairs. In a short while, there were four or five calendars in use.

Over the same period, the desk book version evolved into a detailed diary in which she recorded more information than could ever be needed. She became so meticulous that if she had a nine o'clock appointment and she didn't get in to see the doctor until 9:20, the time had to be changed and sometimes she added the details of what she had done during the twenty minutes she had to wait.

I maintain my own calendar, which by definition is accurate for both of us at all times, since I make all of Mona's appointments and her transportation is my responsibility. However, I felt no need to synchronize mine with Mona's calendar. I must admit that occasionally I neglected to tell Mona when an appointment was changed, but sometimes I did tell her and she didn't record the change.

Eventually there arose the need for correlation among Mona's calendars. Unfortunately, Mona could not grasp the concept of establishing one calendar as a master, with all others synchronized to it. Instead, Mona believed that whatever one she had in front of her was accurate and was frustrated because she was always sure the others were all wrong. Making them all the same became an obsession.

Mona began to lose interest in the calendars in late 2003, although I bought her a new book and pocket version for 2004. I did not buy one in 2005 and she did not notice. However, she still has the old ones and consults them regularly.

The extension of the calendars was a plethora of notes affixed in virtually every available space. Many of these were appropriate and useful, although they represented a maintenance problem in some cases. Now the notes have begun to disappear because she is rapidly losing her ability to write, or even sign her name.

During the period when she was aggressively keeping calendars and writing notes, she was acutely aware that her memory was diminishing. She seemed determined to delay that process.

She tried to do the "Find the Word" puzzles in the paper and did surprisingly well. Now that interest and ability are gone as well.

Mona is always finding long-stored pictures, which she places on display. The displays constantly change and are ever expanding. To help her remember I tell her who is in the picture and she writes it on the back, but that never stops her from asking me again, often because she doesn't trust the note.

Mona uses other devices to maintain her dwindling database. Each evening she goes through a sort of litany using pictures, starting with our children. She asks where they live, where they went to school, who they married, what they do, who their children are, all about them and when we saw them last.

Then she goes through the Daleys (my sister) and the Swans (her sister) and a number of our friends and neighbors. The questions are always the same and sometimes I anticipate the next one and answer two at once, but that makes her feel bad. It makes me feel bad as well.

If time permits, she may go through the litany a second or even a third time. She is trying very hard and although I know it is fruitless, I still can't resist trying to help.

I can only speculate, but I suspect that Alzheimer's victims have an innate fear of doing something either embarrassing or seen as stupid. Mona exhibits this in a refusal to throw things out.

This coping takes many forms that are perhaps unique to the person. Mona's principal one is an extension of her personality and it sometimes has unintended consequences.

For Mona, her innate sociability and affectionate nature became primary tools. She has always been a very outgoing, friendly and social person. One might expect that her Alzheimer's would diminish those traits because of uncertainty, confusion and depression. In her case, they sometimes seem enhanced.

That is particularly true with children, especially babies, toddlers and pre-schoolers. She will often literally squeal with delight at the sight of them. However, whereas previously her next actions were appropriate she has lost those inhibitions, especially with babies. She tends to rush to them with open arms, even as if to pick them up if they are in a stroller or similar conveyance.

If someone is holding the child, Mona approaches as she would to take the baby. In today's world that is not always welcomed by watchful parents. I am constantly alert to that situation and try to either intervene or do my best to allay the fears of an anxious mother or father.

Mona has also become extremely appreciative of those who she sometimes senses are people trying to help her, even when they really aren't. People who speak to her at church always get the same response, a hug and often a kiss regardless of how well she knows or last saw them.

The Visiting Nurse and the Home Health Care Aide get the full treatment, as does the startled mailman if he brings an oversized package or a letter needing a signature to the door and the drivers who take her to Day Care and bring her home. This last group includes a range of people in about equal numbers from young black single mothers working an extra job to make ends meet to older white retired men trying to keep busy and active. The two segments seem to enjoy the interaction equally and invariably Mona invites the one who brought her home to stay for dinner.

Her doctor always gets a kiss hello and goodbye, but in between there is an anomaly. It is as if Mona is completely disinterested in what is going on. The doctor and I discuss her condition and her regression candidly, never using euphemisms to obscure reality. Mona does not participate and often does not seem to hear us. When we leave, she never asks me any questions.

Strangely, there is a different pattern when we visited her Psychiatrist in connection with the Clinical Trials. She always seems to appreciate the attention he provides. However, he does not get a kiss either on arrival or on departure. Not even a hug.

In contrast to this behavior, Mona often overtly uses old facial expressions and body language to convey her criticism of people we are with to me. That can be embarrassing if they don't know the situation.

The three youngest of our granddaughters live nearby. I am not sure that Mona really understands who they are, but she always greets them warmly. While she still had some ability to carry on a conversation, she would make a valiant effort to engage them.

The eldest, Chelsea worked part-time while she was in high school at the Rochester Museum and Science Center. There were some times when she needed a ride home and I agreed to provide it. I always took Mona with me.

When Chelsea would come out of the building, Mona would get excited and as soon as Chelsea was in the car, the litany would begin. "Now where do you live?" "Is it a nice house?" "Do you go to school?" "What grade are you in?" "Do you like school?" "Do you know I taught high school?" Then Mona would start again at the beginning.

To her credit and because of the kind of person she is, Chelsea would pleasantly answer each question, usually in a slightly different way each time always adding a new detail, rather than becoming terser. When we dropped Chelsea off she and Mona would share a hug and a kiss. Then, as we drove away, Mona would ask, "Isn't she a lovely girl?" How could I not agree?

Behaviors which are related more to loss of Executive Function than memory

An early revelation was that memory loss is not the only problem and often not the most important. The more serious is the loss of Executive Function, which is just a fancy term for figuring out how to do something that we remember we want to do.

I suspect that this is the most vexing aspect for the victim. After all, most people forget an occasional name, place or event. However, there is something more frightening about not being able to carry out a fundamental task, which you know that you have done easily, thousands of times.

I can best explain this with a few examples.

When I first began to work again from our home, Mona would often ask me if she could help me in some way. One of the first times she asked me that, I was doing a mailing to about a hundred people and welcomed some assistance. The mailing consisted of individually addressed letters, together with a couple enclosures. I set her up at a table and arranged the envelopes, letters, enclosures and stamps in the proper sequence. Mona understood the task, but I wrote down the steps she had to follow anyway.

I checked with Mona frequently and she was clearly having problems. Each time I did that, I also asked her if she understood what it was that I wanted her to do. Mona told me without hesitation that she was supposed to fold the letters in a particular way, make sure the name on the letter was the same as that on the envelope, fold and insert the enclosures, seal the letters, stamp them and put a rubber band around groups of twenty finished envelopes.

After a couple of hours, Mona said, with tears in her eyes, that she was exhausted and was going to bed. She had done fewer than twenty letters and had not sealed or stamped any of them because she was afraid they weren't right. Ironically, she had done them all correctly. A by-product of a diminished Executive Function is a loss of confidence.

It took me less than an hour to complete the job. Within a matter of a few more months, she became unable to handle inserting an unaddressed one-page newsletter alone in an envelope without great stress.

The same sort of thing happens even when the victim chooses the task and/or initiates the activity.

Whenever the weather is nice Mona wants to be outside, but her drive to be busy if not necessarily productive, leaves little time to enjoy the sun. We have a great number of trees in our yard including two very large weeping willows, so are were always sticks and small branches for Mona to pick up.

Mona's method of doing this however, was an entirely random "target of opportunity" approach, looking for the largest piece she could see, picking it up, scanning for another and so forth, crisscrossing the yard many times, until she tired and quit. The result was that yard always looked as it had before she started.

She also faced the dilemma of how to dispose of the brush that filled her arms. The accepted method was to pile it as neatly as possible at the side of the road, where the Town picks it up regularly except during the winter months. With a hundred foot frontage interrupted only by an eighteen-foot wide driveway, she had a number of equally viable options.

Almost without exception however, her choice would be the five-foot space between the end of the driveway and the mailbox. If she had more than would fit there, she continued on the other side of the mailbox. It mattered not to Mona that on the other side of the driveway she had more than sixty feet of road front before reaching our neighbor's lot line.

Our mailman did not like this arrangement. For the most part he tolerated it, but on a few occasions when the brush pile exceeded his idea of what was acceptable, instead of our mail we would find a printed notice in our box detailing the Post Office Regulation requiring unimpeded access to the box.

This is not to say that Mona always put the yard debris next to the mailbox. If it were late Tuesday afternoon and I had already put the trash barrels out in anticipation of their pick up around 7:00 AM Wednesday, she might put the brush into any partially filled barrel and pile the rest on top of the full barrels.

The trash company workers didn't like this intrusion on their space any more than the mailman did and they expressed their displeasure in different ways.

Now, if the garage door happened to be open while Mona was foraging, everything could end up in there, which wasn't so bad because although she would put it in the trash barrels that made it easier for me to take it out to the roadside. Of course, I had to keep constantly aware of the Town's brush pick-up schedule that for some reason changed often, because if the brush stayed out there too long, Mona would either move it to the mailbox or bring it back in.

However, the worst choice she could make from my perspective was to bring whatever she had gathered in the front door and put it in the kitchen trash receptacle. That was a common occurrence, unfortunately.

Alzheimer's had left Mona with the understanding that some things had to be thrown out and others recycled, but it robbed her of the ability to determine how to do that. Although I constantly searched for out-of-the-way places to put the

Recycle Box, if Mona found it she would always just dump it into the trash barrel.

In fact, if I had taken the trash barrels and Recycle Box out to the road and I didn't watch her carefully, she would go out, dump the recyclable material in the trash barrel and bring the box back in.

There is an ironic corollary to Mona's activities related to yard debris, trash and recycling. Just as Alzheimer's left Mona with the understanding that some things had to be discarded, it also left her with the knowledge that some things should be saved. In this case, it robbed her of the ability to make a decision.

One might conclude that with this condition, Mona would keep everything and that is not the case. However, there developed a list of things that she just would *never* throw out and in some ways, there appeared to be some logic to it.

There was a range to that list, divided into two types.

The first was food, especially small amounts of food. Years ago I used to kid Mona about her habit while cleaning up after dinner of eating those last spoonfuls of food in serving dishes, as if that were some form of conservation. It was probably the memory of a Depression Era mother insisting on cleaning up her plate while thinking of starving children far away. I always thought that was a cruel theory.

She would respond that either there wasn't enough for her lunch the next day, or for the two of us to have for another meal. Now Alzheimer's had taken away her ability to project those outcomes or to remember how she compensated. Consequently, we began to have spoonfuls of things put away in the refrigerator in coffee cups covered with plastic wrap and larger, hopefully dry portions of later unidentifiable things in foil wrappers. Usually both types lost their identity and edibility before anyone thought to retrieve and eat them.

This confused thought process extended to the last few drops of salad dressing in plastic bottles, hardly enough to cover a small lettuce leaf. Since there clearly was not enough for another use, she bought a new bottle. This led inevitably to an abundance of salad dressing bottles, sometimes exceeding a dozen, accumulating in the refrigerator. Periodically, our daughter Maryellen or I would arbitrarily throw them all out.

However, Mona had another "rationale" for keeping the salad dressing bottles. It was the bottles themselves. She just knew that one day she would need them for something. She would retrieve them, wash them out, remove the labels and put them on a shelf in the garage. Periodically they went back into the trash barrel. Mona never noticed.

Actually, Mona never saw a container she didn't like, especially if it were made of plastic. She hid them away until no one remembered what they had once held. I was always pleased, however at how many things for which I had long been searching that I would find during my periodic sweeps through containers ranging from peanut butter jars to coffee cans, all washed and with labels either removed or covered. I won't even discuss pizza and Krispy Kreme Donut boxes.

However, the largest and most inexplicable cache was always the cardboard cores of toilet tissue and paper towel rolls. For Mona these items seemed a mission. If they went in the trash, she retrieved them. If I bent them in half, I would be the recipient of a withering stare. Peculiarly, I would occasionally find a paper towel core, with one or two others forced inside it. I never have figured that out.

Finally, I must talk about zip lock bags, perhaps Mona's favorite container. They were the only containers that she really tried to re-use. She turned them inside out and washed them, but seemed unaware that it was often very difficult to get them clean. Fortunately, her method of drying them was to carefully stand them up on the kitchen counter, making it easy for me to gather them up and properly dispose of them.

Eventually all Alzheimer's victims lose the ability to dress themselves, but first comes the loss of an ability to decide what to put on. Sometimes victims introduce new "logic" that often has little to do with the decision. This was the first indication of Mona having a problem with dressing.

Within a few miles of our house are three Catholic Churches. Although all three are essentially located on a seven-mile stretch of the same road, Mona thinks of them as fundamentally different, and over time that perception has become stronger, not weaker.

The choice of which to attend depends mostly on scheduling convenience. On Sunday morning if I tell Mona that we are going to Mass soon, the first question is where.

If I say St. Catherine's because their 10:30 Mass is the next one available, she will head off to get dressed. If she takes too long to get ready, making it obvious that we will be late, and I tell her that instead we are going to St. Louis at 11:00, she will immediately disappear to change her clothes. If that takes too long as well and the choice becomes 11:30 at Transfiguration, she will make another change. Sometimes the change is as subtle as shoes.

As I write this, Mona is beginning to have more difficulty with dressing, although I resist the temptation to give her more assistance than she really needs. When there is no urgency, I leave her on her own. This sometimes results in strange combinations, but she handles the basic tasks, including still double tying her sneakers.

Occasionally, Mona will bring me alternatives and ask me to choose. I resist doing that as long as I can, but if I sense that she is getting upset, I tell her what to put on. Sometimes she does it. Sometimes she ignores the advice. Or she forgets it.

On days when she goes to Day Care, one of us has an appointment, or we are heading for church I act as a coach in the process laying out the clothes I think she should wear. Sometimes that confuses her and she doesn't know what to put on first, but gentle suggestions get her past that.

Two things are interesting to me in this process. She has no problem putting on her bra, using the upside down, inside out and backward method. Additionally, she not only always makes sure to put her orthotics in her shoes, she can lace the shoes when necessary, and with great facility, she ties them always adding that double knot for security.

There is another behavior related to this impaired Executive Function. In effect, it is the corollary and can be more serious or at least more annoying. Mona is not able to project the consequences of an action she is about to take.

For example, she closes the doors to all rooms at all times. In its most benign consequence, one must always put down anything one is carrying in order to open the door. In its most vexing, one runs into doors in the dark.

She may change the existing location of any movable object, which she may encounter, with its new location nearly always being out of sight. By the same lack of logic, toilet paper rolls may become part of the décor in any room. The exception to that rule is the bathroom.

Behaviors not directly related to impaired memory

Other behaviors emerge in an Alzheimer's victim that do not appear directly related to the loss of memory or to coping with that loss. They also are not related to the loss of Executive Function. While perplexing, they are not usually worrisome.

This is probably an appropriate time to discuss the significant changes in Mona's sleep patterns during the course of her Alzheimer's Disease. Prior to developing Alzheimer's her sleep patterns were stable. She was usually asleep by midnight and awakened around seven the next morning, with rare exception.

As the Alzheimer's progressed, that changed. For many years, we had routinely gone to bed following the eleven o'clock local TV news. Now, suddenly one evening Mona would announce that she wasn't going to bed. The first time it happened, I just went up, figuring that she would soon follow. However, that didn't happen.

In the morning, I would find her wide-awake sitting in the recliner watching television and not acting the least bit tired. I would get her ready for Day Care and off she'd go, arriving home that evening as chipper as when she left. Often this would happen two nights in a row and rarely but sometimes, a third.

A variation of this was that occasionally she would go to bed at the usual time on the first night, but get up within an hour and go downstairs.

Sometimes Mona simply returned to her normal sleep routine. On other occasions, she might sleep for extended periods of twenty-four to thirty-six or more hours eating little or nothing.

During this period, Mona was in the "Nursing Home Without Walls Program" administered by the Visiting Nurse Service. The program included Day Care, Home Health Care Aide assistance and a bi-weekly check-up by a Registered Visiting Nurse.

The first time Mona pulled an "all-nighter", I reported it to the Visiting Nurse. Her reply was, "Well there was a full moon". I laughed and expressed my disbelief of such things. The Nurse just said, "Lots of people think as you do, but most Nurses will tell you there is something to it".

The second time it happened I again reported it to the Nurse. She asked if there had been a full moon. I said I had no idea. Without a word, she picked up the newspaper and handed it to me. There was a full moon.

A few weeks later, when the Nurse arrived she asked with a bit of a twinkle in her eye, how Mona had slept the night before. I told her Mona had stayed up all night and asked how she knew that. She said there was a full moon.

It didn't happen every time the moon was full, but every time it did happen, it was during the phase of a full moon. I checked it out on the Internet and there is a lot of support for the full moon theory, but I have never heard a doctor say that.

There is also a great deal of support, even among doctors for something called "Sundowning Syndrome". According to this theory, many Dementia victims suffer behavioral changes somewhat regularly within a few hours before and after sunsets. They become agitated, upset and sometimes belligerent including shouting. I saw some evidence of that with Mona, but not with enough frequency or intensity for it to be conclusive.

In Mona's case, her bizarre sleep patterns while of mild concern were not a big issue. She was not a wanderer so there was little chance of her deciding to go for a walk in the middle of the night. Besides, Tipper was in her kennel in the kitchen. If Mona had opened a door and gone out, Tipper would undoubtedly have done what she always did: raise a great ruckus until she got my attention and I came downstairs to remedy the situation.

Another example of behavior that is perplexing, though not particularly worrisome appears when we are eating away from home. That activity had always been part of our life together, whether it was on a trip, at the club to which we belonged, a local restaurant, at parties or privately with friends or family. Our choice of the venue depended upon, as Mona often said, whether we were "going out to eat" or "dining out".

After Mona began to suffer more of the debilitations of Alzheimer's the number of times we "went out to eat" decreased significantly. This was simply because instead of being easier than staying home it became more difficult, principally because I had to get two of us ready to go.

The frequency of "dining out" experiences also diminished because frankly we were invited fewer places and from my standpoint, "dining out" on birthdays and anniversaries was mostly to give Mona a break from the task of preparing dinner. Now, since I was doing all the cooking I usually just elected to prepare something a little special at home.

While ordering a meal in a restaurant was a bit problematic for Mona, eating it was usually not. However, she began to develop some behaviors, with which I had to become more vigilant. For example, if I weren't paying attention she would eat all the bread in the basket while waiting for dinner because she didn't remember that I had ordered dinner for her.

If dinner were a buffet, despite my best efforts, she would take large portions of absolutely everything on the buffet, resulting in a plate twice as full as that of anyone else. As she became satisfied, she would slow down, but when everyone else had finished she would adamantly refuse to surrender her plate and keep eating long after anyone else.

At a plated meal, she developed an end-of-meal routine, which I believe was from an early life experience that we both had, but not together. There was a wonderful Italian family restaurant on the north side of Syracuse, called Bersani's. The food was great, the portions large and the price right. In those Depression Days, a full spaghetti and meatball dinner was sixty-five cents.

Both Mona's parents and mine took us to Bersani's whenever they had the sixty-five cents.

My father always told us that the way you could tell a good Italian restaurant was if Italians ate there. By that measure, Bersani's was a great restaurant. There were always many Italian families there enjoying the food and as much Italian as English was spoken.

It was common at that restaurant when the family had finished eating for them to pass their plates to the mother, who would scrape what remained onto her plate, commenting often when someone had not eaten all of one thing or another. She would then stack the scraped plates, placing her plate of scraps on the top ready for removal.

When our children were old enough to eat at the table, Mona often used that same routine at home when we were finished.

As her Alzheimer's advanced, Mona did not quite do as the mothers in Bersani's did, but she had her own, similar routine. To begin with, she would eat everything. Then she would wipe the plate clean either with a remaining piece of bread or her napkin. If something sticky remained, she would pour a little water from her glass or even a little coffee on the plate and scrub until it was clean. Then she'd do the silverware.

If I could head off that behavior, I would. If not, I would try to catch the eye of a server and quietly ask that he or she remove the plate and silver.

Very unexpected and among the most frustrating of the effects of Dementia is the matter of obsessive behavior. I am sure that the root of that lies in the feeling of the victims that they are losing control and can help themselves by getting better organized. However, it is so pervasive that I suspect its cause is even more likely the loss of another mental inhibition.

This takes several forms (arranging, repackaging, maintenance), each with its own effect on others. In some sense, the Carekeeper contributes to this activity by putting up little signs about what, when or how to do things. That gives the victim the impression that order will somehow overcome the chaos he or she feels. Nevertheless, in the process, it can also change the behavior of the Carekeeper and that is not necessarily a good thing.

The most benign of this type of activity is arranging things. For the most part this is a harmless activity except when you are watching it. Then it can drive you up the wall. I have just learned to look in a different direction when it is in progress.

Mona has several hundred cookbooks accumulated over forty years, most of which were on shelves in the family room. They have always been a source of great pride and even greater comfort to Mona.

One time I suggested that she develop an index of favorite recipes on the computer. However, Mona demonstrated to me many times that if she needed a recipe or if someone asked her about one, she could walk to the shelves and select the book that included that specific recipe.

She would often take a book from the shelf and read it through as one would a novel. She could also look at the wall and tell if a book were out of place or missing. If someone had put a book back in the wrong place, within minutes Mona would notice and move it.

I had always accepted that as rather normal. However, now Mona arranges and rearranges the books and the pictures that share their shelves, sometimes several nights in a row. Mona also rearranges appliances in the kitchen sometimes by size and sometimes by color. On occasion, she searches for and brings out some little or never used appliances to complete a display, or hides an often-used one, causing a search the next time I need it.

I can do the grocery shopping in less than half the time by myself and I usually plan my trips accordingly. However, I always take her if I need to go when she is around and wants to go.

We have the same deal we used to have with our children. If you can't find me, go to the front door and wait, but do not go outside. That works very well, because Mona walks so slowly looking at everything as if she had never seen it before, and of course, she constantly arranges the merchandise on the shelves.

There used to be a joke about a man whose wife was so neat that if he got up to go to the bathroom in the middle of the night, she'd make the bed. Mona is approaching that.

Often this kind of activity causes additional work. If I come in from outside, even if I tell her that I intend to go back out in a few minutes, when I take my coat off it will be immediately hung up. The trouble is it can be in any closet in the house.

If I kick off my shoes when I sit down, Mona will quickly pick them up, take them into the front hall and line them up at the foot of the stairs. Instead of just being able to slip into them when I get up, I have to find them. They are always heels against the wall, so I still can't slip them on.

Trivial, indeed, and perhaps whiney, but with no pun intended, you don't walk in my shoes. It is just one more aspect of this frustrating disease.

Arranging things has nothing to do with putting them where they belong. It does have to do with getting them out of sight or at least into some kind of display. That leads to dirty pans, left to soak before washing, ending up in the oven. It also leads to endless searches for utensils, dishes, food, and just about anything else you need.

Then there are the booby traps. When you have finally located that two-quart saucepan that you were looking for on the top shelf of the cupboard with the good dishes, be very careful when you take it down. It may have some of the dishes it replaced in it, ready to crash to the floor. On the other hand, it may be full of that open bag of rice you were looking for days earlier. That one took me weeks to clean up.

Repackaging is another constant activity and a double-edged sword. We have a good-sized refrigerator, with an icemaker that allows Mona to repackage her favorite cider into ice cube trays.

I buy milk by the gallon. As soon as we use some of the milk Mona repackages the remainder into something smaller, maybe even a two-quart measuring cup with Saran Wrap stretched across the top. Each time the milk is used that process continues using smaller and smaller containers. The problem is that when it is in a small Tupperware box, it stops looking like milk and usually ends up becoming sour and thrown out.

To complete the process, Mona washes the jug, fills it with tap water and puts it back in the refrigerator or worse yet the freezer. One day last winter I removed five jugs of frozen water and several bags of ice cubes from the freezer and dumped them out. Of course, I had to thaw the jugs first. That will raise the blood pressure.

By maintenance, I mean obsessively doing ordinary tasks such as washing dishes, setting the table, wiping down cupboards and counter tops. However, often Mona doesn't really get things clean. She collects dishes and silverware in the sink to wash, but if there is even a small distraction before that is completed a problem arises.

Returning to the task, Mona often assumes that she washed them and puts them away. I wash more things coming out of the cupboards than Mona does before she puts them in. To make it easier, I apply no judgment and wash everything *before* I use it. I try to ignore the expressions on people's faces when I remove all the dishes for dinner from the cupboard and proceed to wash them.

The subject of maintenance also highlights another phenomenon. There seem to be some things that an Alzheimer's victim remembers, but one wishes they would forget. One of the three toilets in our house developed a defective gasket and when flushed it would not refill. By the time I fixed it, Mona had developed the habit of filling the tank by hand using a bucket. That was, of course, helpful for a short period.

However, Mona did two things that were total wastes of time. The first was that she thought that all three toilets had the problem. The second was to develop the habit of flushing the toilet and immediately taking the top off the tank to look. Finding it empty, Mona began hauling water to fill the tank. Weeks later, long after I made the repair she was still doing it.

A less onerous thing is that Mona eats all the time and has definitely forgotten her mother's warning that she will spoil her dinner. She loves sweets, especially ice cream. If I buy two half gallons of ice cream and don't hide them, they will both be gone in sixteen hours without me eating a spoonful. By the way, she repackages the ice cream constantly sometimes into zip lock bags so you can never tell how much is left. She loves zip lock bags.

Mona had always been a TV watcher and although her tastes varied, there was a constant thread. She liked complicated stories, which was also true of her reading tastes. It always amazed me that she was as comfortable with an afternoon soap opera as a book by Clancy, Ludlum or Grisham. She had no time for half-hour sitcoms or the steady stream of agony TV described as "self help". That has changed dramatically.

At first, as her memory loss began to affect her attention span, Mona began to watch things like Jerry Springer and Ricki Lake and game shows when I wasn't in the room. If sitcoms were relatively mindless, but with lots of action, she would try that but became unable to handle an hour-long drama, especially if it had an ensemble cast and multiple story lines.

For a while, Mona was into cable news shows, grasping at what I'm sure she thought was a connection to what was happening in the world around her. Nonetheless, the September 11, 2001 attack on the World Trade Center was beyond her comprehension and marked a major change in her.

She kept interpreting re-runs of the attacks as new events. Even today, she will call me when one of those planes crashes into the Tower. She reacts as though it was just happening and she was seeing it live. That was five years ago.

Not able to keep things in context, Mona became unable to determine what is important and what was not and acronyms began to bother her terribly. Several times each evening she would ask what CNN, MSNBC, SARS, WTC, WMD and a host of others meant. Sometimes she would ask what FOX stands for. It is difficult to answer that one on several levels.

Technology has further complicated things. Since Mona finds the discussions difficult to follow, while I'm watching the discussion she is reading the crawl across the bottom of the screen and asking me questions about that. Often by the time, she gets the question out the subject on the crawl that captured her attention has moved off the screen, so I can't help her and she has forgotten what she wanted to know anyway.

Another unexpected aspect, far less frustrating, is the constant wonder at "new" things or experiences. Except for their repetition, these are good things and the joy they produce is well worth the annoyance.

The sight of a bright red Cardinal nestled in the green grass of the back yard causes such great excitement, that it warrants running upstairs to ask me to share. The wonderment each night at how dark it is when all the lights in the neighborhood are out is definitely sincere. The exit each Sunday at the beginning of Mass by the children four to seven years old to a nearby classroom for Sunday school always evokes a comment and sometimes a tear. Since she does not remember these events, they are ever new.

Mona also developed a strong belief that anything that is broken is repairable if taken to someone. Mona does not limit her vigilance to those things under her normal purview. She goes through my office wastebaskets, retrieves empty printer ink cartridges, and returns them to the supply shelf. When she replaces a light bulb, she puts away the bad one along with the good ones.

Periodically, packed suitcases appear by the front door. One time I checked and the suitcase was full of summer clothes. It was September and the weather was still warm. I left the suitcase in the hall. A couple of weeks later, the weather turned dramatically colder and concurrently, some of her warmer clothes disappeared. She had changed her traveling wardrobe. However, I don't believe either of us knew her planned destination.

Obviously during the time she has had Alzheimer's many external things have happened that Mona not only does not remember, but that she also has not been able to comprehend. One in particular was sad for me personally.

In October 2006, I fulfilled a sixty-year-old dream that began when I was in high school with the publishing of my first book, "The Compliant, Curious and Critical Catholic". I was very proud of that accomplishment and, naturally wanted to share my delight with Mona.

When I received the first copies of the book, I waited for just the right moment when she was both relaxed and not distracted to hand her a copy. Mona took it, silently looked it over for a minute or so and then handed it back saying, "It's pretty". She left it on my desk, busied herself with other things and then went downstairs. I was crestfallen.

The next day she came into my office and after a while, she picked up the book from where she had left it asking if she could look at it. Of course, I said she could and she left the room. A few minutes later, she returned and pointing to my name on the front cover in type a half inch high said, "Did you see this?"

I said I had and she said, "That's nice" and left with the book. A little later, she returned with the book, this time pointing to my picture on the back cover. "Is that you?" she asked. I said yes and elatedly she replied, "I thought it was!" She left again.

In addition to my picture, the back cover had a short biography and a brief summary of the book, but she didn't notice that. However, on her next visit, she excitedly had something new to ask whether I had seen. It was her name in the Dedication. That really pleased her.

As the days, weeks and months went by periodically I would find Mona's copy of my book and page through it. The first hundred pages or so are largely biographical and apparently, every time she came across a name or a place she recognized she underlined or circled it, but she never mentioned it to me again. However, she never got past about thirty pages probably because she always started again from the beginning. I don't believe she has ever comprehended that I wrote it.

That was disappointing. Heartbreaking, actually.

She won't know about this one either.

Behaviors Common to Alzheimer's Disease not yet exhibited

Recently, there has been some interesting new information in the national press regarding the viability of a new test for Alzheimer's Disease. It is suspected that an early indication of the disease is the loss of the sense of smell related to certain specific and common odors.

While I was editing this chapter, the following appeared in Newsday:

> "The inability to identify 10 everyday smells—from smoke to soap—can be used to predict Alzheimer's Disease, scientists have discovered.
> The smell test was as effective at diagnosis as a memory test, and was better than a brain scan.
> The findings by D.P. Devanand, a professor of clinical psychiatry and neurology at Columbia Presbyterian Medical Center, were presented this week at the annual American College of Neuro-pharmacology meeting in San Juan, Puerto Rico.
> Scientists have known for more than a decade that the brain's smell center is hard-hit in Alzheimer's, but using smell tests to diagnose the disease has never caught on. Devanand has been testing the predictive value of a 40-item smell test developed by Richard Doty of the University of Pennsylvania.
> In the latest study, 150 patients ranging in age from 43 to 85 with mild to moderate memory problems, and 63 healthy volunteers were asked to identify 40 odors on scratch cards.
> Most normal people scored between 35 and 40. People in the earliest stages of Alzheimer's, before cognitive difficulty renders them unable to understand the exercise, scored in the 20s.
> More recently, researchers have narrowed the test to the smells that best predicted Alzheimer's. Inability to identify smoke topped the list. The others

were menthol, leather, lilac, pineapple, soap, strawberry, natural gas, lemon and clove. Devanand said he is not sure why these smells are more often lost to memory impairment."

I found this article to be particularly interesting because long before I became convinced that Mona was suffering from Alzheimer's, I had noticed that Mona did not have as acute a sense of smell as I do or as she once had. On a couple of occasions when she was still doing some of the cooking Mona would put oil in a pan to heat or bread in a toaster, sit down and not notice when it began to smoke even though she was right there in the room. That is one of the common odors cited and is one of the reasons why she does not cook any more.

There are two other effects of Alzheimer's about which I was not aware until I attended a seminar presented by our local Alzheimer's Association. The leader said Alzheimer's victims often suffer related diminished hearing and reduced peripheral vision. As if, they don't have enough problems.

Some time before, I had started to notice that when I came downstairs from my office for some reason during the day, I would startle Mona as I walked in the room. I assumed that was because she had forgotten that I was there and that is definitely a part of it. Then I began to notice that she wouldn't even look up until I was quite close.

I am sure that all three of these symptoms are related to Alzheimer's, but I don't believe that it necessarily means that every victim actually loses the sense of smell, hearing or vision. It may merely mean that they are unable to process the new information because they can't handle the subtlety of the source not being readily visible. However, in the end what difference does that make?

Probably the two questions people ask me most often are: "Does Mona wander off?" and "Does she get violent sometimes?" My answer to both is no and if it were not, the issue of my ability to care for her would be in serious question. Those are dramatic conditions, requiring specific responses.

If the first question were: Could Mona go from Point A to Point B unaided or more important, could she find her way back to Point A the answer would be no. I suspect that the reason many of those people wander off is not that they intended to do so but that they don't realize that they can't navigate alone.

Mona still understands that distinction. One summer day, I saw that clearly. I took Mona to get her hair cut by a woman who has cut it for her for more than thirty years. The shop is on the second floor of a two-story building. However, since they built the structure into a hillside, the back door is at ground level. I always drive around back to drop her off.

The back door is not marked. This time, when I pulled up to the door that Mona has entered unaided, several hundred times she asked me where to go and when I told her, she asked me to show her. Mona may reach the point of wandering, but she is not there yet.

I had been aware that wandering was a problem with some Alzheimer's victims. Actually, I thought it was with all of them. However, I did not know that they sometimes become violent and physically abusive.

Although I have seen Mona frustrated with her condition, angry at her diminished abilities and sad with her lot I have never seen any evidence of a tendency to violence. That would be very troubling to me because I am a very non-violent person and I'm not sure how I would deal with violence from Mona. I guess I had better give that some thought.

One day, Mona's Home Health Care Aide told me that I have given her feelings of guilt regarding her father who died recently of Alzheimer's after several years in a Nursing Home. She feels that way because she perceives that her father was much more functional when he moved to the Nursing Home that Mona is. Yet, she sees that Mona is thriving.

The Aide now feels that her decision to institutionalize her father may have been premature. I think that one must do what one feels is right and then not entertain any regret.

Mona has exhibited one other inexplicable behavior for nearly as long as I have thought she had Dementia. When she sits, she thinks the floor is vibrating beneath her feet. At first Mona talked about it just when she was sitting in her usual chair in our family room but now it is wherever she sits, whether at home or elsewhere.

I have no theory about that one and I don't think I will spend any time trying to develop one. The doctors I have told about this completely ignore it.

CHAPTER 8

▼

USING AVAILABLE
SERVICES AND CREATIVE
CARE STRATEGIES

I am virtually certain that scholars have studied the psychology of the Carekeeper. However, I for one have no interest in reading about it or even trying to learn about their conclusions.

Although I admit to the fact that I do not know all the answers, I consider myself mature, more than minimally educated and possessed of sufficient judgment to have arrived at this point in my life reasonably unscathed. I also believe that although I have described the Carekeeping of an Alzheimer's victim as "the ultimate do-it-yourself-project", most of it yields to common sense.

NIKE has a slogan, which seems appropriate to this situation and many others: "Just Do It!"

Nonetheless, I will readily admit that one can easily fall into the trap of following that advice too literally. One person cannot do everything. Perhaps the better admonition is "Just Get It Done!" Accept the resources that are available and don't feel guilty about using them.

At first, I felt that this was my job and mine alone and I needed to figure out how to do it all. I did not realize that the task of the Carekeeper was really to manage in detail the living of two lives. Daunting as it may appear, reality further exacerbates that task in that the victim is constantly making it more difficult by illogical behavior. In addition to the work involved, there is frustration, anger and depression to manage.

The Carekeeper needs help to "Just Get It Done!"

There are two parts to this chapter. In the first, I will discuss the available outside assistance that I have found to be worthwhile. In the second, I will provide some creative strategies to deal with the illogical behavior of the victim, the frustration it produces, the anger it elicits and the attendant depression.

However, do not expect a detailed guide to success. This is what works for me. Take what you can use, but don't stop "Just Getting It Done!" in whatever way you can. Your way may be better.

The first thing to be remembered in considering the use of outside services is to avoid being self-righteous. Often these services are offered simply as benefits to the Carekeeper and they certainly are, but in fact they usually benefit the victim as well, even if secondarily.

If one is of Irish descent as I am, or otherwise given to guilt it is easy to interpret such services and assistance, as "these are things you can do if you are not really up to the task". This is the "real men don't eat quiche" syndrome and I initially dismissed these ideas as giving in to weakness.

Examples of such services are Home Health Care Aides, Adult Day Care, Transportation Services, Respite Care, Support Groups and Seminars. Not all are for everyone, but my real concern was that Mona would reject any of these things out of hand. That was a basic miscalculation because I was thinking in terms of the pre-Alzheimer's Mona.

Home Health Care Aides do what the name implies and much more. They have sufficient training, but are not Registered Nurses and they work by the hour. Early on, I ran into problems with getting Mona to take regular showers. I really feel that this issue was mostly her effort to assert her independence and right to decide for herself when she would bathe or shower.

The situation had reached the point that the mention of the subject made her completely intransigent. I needed to either resort to physical force or get help. Since the former is not part of my nature, I chose the latter.

Over the years, Mona has been in the hospital enough times to accept the discipline of hospital routine. On the two days a week the Home Health Care Aide comes to the house, she arrives while Mona is still asleep. The Aide and I enter the bedroom together, with me carrying Mona's daily medications and a glass of water. I wake Mona telling her that the Aide is here and insisting that she sit up on the edge of the bed to take the medicine.

Then although she doesn't need my help, I give her a hand to stand up and suggest that she go into the bathroom. As soon as she does, the Aide makes the bed to establish that Mona is up for the day, and I leave the room. When Mona has finished using the toilet, the Aide enters the bathroom with a towel and clean clothes and the shower becomes a fait accompli.

If there is time left in the hour and the weather is nice, the Aide may take Mona for a short walk or they just chat for a few minutes. One spring day Mona and the Aide planted some flowers, which gave them an activity for several months. We created an environment in which Mona would accept direction and I had one less thing to worry about.

I had not expected this reaction, but sometimes Mona genuinely seems to enjoy having the Aide around. I think it is because the Aide is very gentle and very attentive. Mona enjoys being fussed over in a way that perhaps I don't.

I had greater misgivings about Adult Day Care, plus considerably more guilt. It was recommended by both Mona's Primary Care Physician and her Psychiatrist, but it seemed to me that the emphasis was on "giving me a break" at Mona's expense. I even recall referring to Day Care in an e-mail to the family as "warehousing" Mona so I could play and said I would never do that.

Her doctor recommended Day Care when Mona returned from Conifer Park, long before she showed evidence of Alzheimer's. I took her to a center nearby to see what they had to offer. As I opened the door, Mona took one look inside, burst into tears and headed back to the car. On the way home, she begged me to promise her that she would never have to go to such a place. It took me ten years before I considered it again.

Every Monday, Wednesday and Friday Mona goes to an Adult Day Care Center about five miles away, from nine-thirty in the morning until four-thirty in the afternoon. It is a small center in a local church, with ten to fifteen attendees and a staff of three. She gets a Continental breakfast, a catered hot lunch, an afternoon snack and much love and attention.

They have a full schedule of activities every day and sometimes go on field trips, one of which was a boat ride on the Erie Canal. Mona has no recollection of what she has done all day, but she has clearly enjoyed her day and she is pleasantly tired when she arrives home.

Although her absence does give me more flexibility in my schedule, I believe the greater benefit is for Mona. She has a chance to socialize with others in similar situations, does things she would not otherwise have the opportunity to do and she gets away from me for a while.

I use outside transportation services only in connection with the Day Care. The drive each morning and afternoon with her fellow participants adds to the feeling of an event. She greets the driver with a smile in the morning and he or she usually gets a hug when they drop her off.

Many things about the care of an Alzheimer's victim are cosmetic, in the sense of the manner in which they happen. I could drive her to and from Day Care but it would not be special and I am sure that it would often be difficult for me to get her into or out of the car. The driver makes it special.

I must say that during the time Mona is gone, I never find myself looking for something to do. I use the time to get haircuts and run errands. I schedule doing the laundry, major grocery shopping, doctors' appointments, car servicing and occasional business meetings for those days.

I also do things around the house, which would be impossible with Mona here, like mopping the kitchen floor, cleaning out closets and putting things away in their proper places. The latter would be nearly a full time job, if I let it.

For those unfamiliar with Respite Care, some Assisted Living Facilities and Nursing Homes provide it as both a marketing strategy and a means of making their vacant rooms produce income. They offer short-term stays separately to non-residents and/or their Carekeepers.

In Mona's case, they would certainly place her in a locked area of the facility with very restricted access to other areas. I am sure that there are instances in which that might be necessary. However, that *does* sound like "warehousing" to me. I realize that it is foolhardy to say never, but I do not expect that we will ever use these services.

I mentioned my feelings about support groups and seminars earlier, but perhaps I should clarify my position. They obviously have value or they would not exist.

I personally do not feel that I get much out of support groups. However, I do find one-on-one conversations with others facing the same or similar situation to be extremely beneficial, whether they are formal or informal. That was, in fact the rationale for this book. Perhaps the problem with support groups is an environmental issue, with the size of the group being inversely proportional to its value.

Alzheimer's is an intensely personal disease for both the victim and the Carekeeper. In that sense, it seems to cry out for privacy, and the "can you top this" style of some support groups is destructive of that. I also do not find wallowing in collective misery to be an effective use of my time. That is not to say that all support groups feature these activities, but finding the right one is difficult and often the quarry is not worth the quest.

I also think the inevitability of the situation divides the group. Some are desperately looking for a miracle for the victim and others sympathy or perhaps praise for themselves. Others are just trying to find ways to get through the experience, providing the best possible care for the victims, while suffering the least damage to themselves. Sometimes in a support group, the former outnumber the latter. That is not productive.

Seminars are a different thing and once again, my personal feelings may be unlike those of most people. I find pressure shortens my attention span. My needs for information about Alzheimer's are very narrow. I want to know about a specific medicine. I want to know if the behavior I see in Mona is typical. The randomness of the disease and its variability militate against that when it comes to seminars designed to satisfy the masses.

I find it more productive to spend time on the Internet looking for a specific answer than to spend the same amount of time waiting for a new nugget of information amid a torrent of material I have heard before. Early in the process, seminars can be quite useful in getting to a comfortable level of knowledge. However, I feel they are of limited real value on an ongoing basis.

How then, does one develop effective strategies for dealing with the multiple aberrant behaviors of the Alzheimer's victim? In answering that gut question, I can only tell you what has been working for me.

First, you have to want to do it. The motivation for wanting to do it, whether it is love, pride, honor, duty, pressure from others, economic or something else, is not important. You do have to want to do it, unconditionally. All I can tell you for sure is that if you do it to write a book, there are easier subjects I could suggest.

Next, you have to be convinced unequivocally, that you *can* do it and survive. "The Little Engine That Could" is a wonderful children's story, but if you are going to chug up *this* mountain, your mantra must be: "You're damn right I can … You're damn right I can" …

Now we come to something quite tricky. One of my most revealing discoveries when I first began to learn about fictional literature, was the concept usually taught in connection with theater, but equally relevant to novels and short stories. It is simply though counter-intuitively defined, as "the willing suspension of disbelief".

This is useful analogously to the Carekeeper in dealing with an Alzheimer's victim. It is critical that you suspend disbelief in certain intuitive beliefs. This will become much clearer, I hope later in this chapter.

After that, you have to have an exit strategy. We hear a lot about exit strategies, but rarely does anyone ever mention that the most important part of that strategy is the definition of the criteria, which trigger its implementation. That is essential in this case, because there inevitably comes a time when your mantra changes to "Hell no, I can't … Hell no, I can't" and that is okay.

Finally, you must find your "cruising speed". Cruising speed is usually defined as the rate as which the vehicle, in this case the Carekeeper, operates most efficiently, optimizing the trade off between fuel consumption and performance.

We each have our own individual cruising speed, which allows us to react smoothly to changes and unexpected events. It may take some experimentation to find it, but then one can turn on the cruise control and not touch it again.

With all these factors in place, you can implement your personal "Triple A Strategy" of Anticipate, Avoid and Accommodate. You will soon find that the key element of this strategy is to learn how to make the disease work <u>for</u> you and not <u>against</u> you.

All planning, whether strategic, tactical or operational, is a process and a way of thinking about things. One is never finished with Anticipating, Avoiding or Accommodating.

Anticipation is a constant activity and the primary defense against potential problems.

Let's look at Anticipation and its principal tool, visualization. About twenty-five years ago my older son, who was far more into computers than I raised the possibility of assigning jobs to volunteers at a professional golf tournament based on a weighted formula that valued their availability more than their preference using a computer. In some ways that flies in the face of the concept of volunteerism, but it can work effectively if it is logical.

There are some inherent difficulties in that proposition, but our immediate problem was to define all the required jobs and to establish their priorities. I gave the task to my son, and in very short order, he discovered that he didn't know how to start. He had attended many tournaments and worked at a few, so he had the basic knowledge required.

I asked him to visualize himself as the first golfer of the day walking onto the first tee. I asked him to imagine looking around and to tell me who and what he saw there. Then he was to decide which of those things we did not need. Once he did that, the task though tedious and time consuming was straightforward.

There is an excellent analogy in that. The best available tool for Anticipating is to visualize, not just the scene and situation, but what might happen while the Alzheimer's victim is present.

Start with a single room and move throughout the house. Don't forget the garage, the basement and the yard. Then expand your horizons to places you and the victim must go, like doctor's visits, church and homes of family and friends.

Every time a new situation arises, make visualization and Anticipation your first exercise, and each time you revisit a situation, review your visualization. Remember that the condition of the victim is far from static. What is an acceptable environment at one time may not remain so.

I have used a wide variety of Avoidance and Accommodation strategies since Mona has had Alzheimer's. Some Accommodation strategies have been effective temporarily, but later I have found it necessary to shift to Avoidance. Sometimes that works in reverse.

An example of shifting from Accommodation to Avoidance had to do with Mona driving. I mentioned earlier that Mona had not driven a car since late 1993. Since she no longer had a valid driver's license, for a while that was sufficient reason for her to not to consider driving. For good measure, I mentioned that our insurance did not cover her although that was admittedly a stretch of the truth.

In other words, I Accommodated the situation of the car being available to her by presenting her with what appeared to be a rational, albeit not totally correct, argument against driving it. However, she had not forgotten how to operate a car, as I discovered one day when I had left it in the driveway and found it in the garage. Her access to the car keys represented a very real risk.

I shifted into the Avoidance mode by discontinuing my practice of leaving my keys on the family room TV and instead placing them in the desk drawer in my office. In a few weeks, it was no longer an issue.

The principal thing I had to remember was that my goal was to allow Mona to continue to live in our home as long as I was able to care for her and maintain her quality of life. All the words in that sentence are equally important.

In order to accomplish that goal, I felt it was necessary to allow Mona to make as many decisions for herself as possible. Although they were less restrictive at the outset and probably will be more restrictive in the future, as I write this, the following are the ground rules affecting Mona's quality of life:

- She can go anywhere in the house, garage and yard, whenever she chooses.

- She can sleep as late as she likes on unless she has a scheduled commitment.

- She can nap when she chooses and she sets her own schedule for it.

- She can snack on anything that is available at any time.

- She can select whatever she wants to wear, subject to my general review.

This level of independence works well and she feels comfortable with it. However, before Mona had Alzheimer's she was a rigorously scheduled person. One of the major effects of the disease, at least in her case is that she now sleeps a lot. As I mentioned earlier, sometimes her sleep patterns get very erratic, but she probably averages twelve hours a day sleeping or napping.

Mona's penchant for sleeping in is an example of how, under certain very specific circumstances, Alzheimer's can work to the Carekeeper's advantage. Left on her own, Mona would rarely awake before eleven. In addition, when she does wake up, she may spend another half hour or more in the bedroom, getting dressed, making the bed and just puttering.

Mona does not wander, she does not have anxiety attacks and she is not confrontational. Therefore, I am comfortable leaving her alone in the house while she is asleep, but I provide a large margin of error for returning before she is up.

I always do some things to make her feel comfortable with that approach. I have three identical signs printed in huge red type on an 8.5 x 11 sheet of paper. I scotch tape one on the mirror in the master bathroom, another on the kitchen counter and a third on the screen of the TV in the family room. They read, "Mona: I have gone to do an errand. I will be back by eleven o'clock. Bob"

Many elements of Mona's life require management and strategies of Avoidance and Accommodation. She has to be up, dressed and ready to go to Day Care by 9:20 AM on Monday, Wednesday and Friday, and Mona has never been one to get up in the morning if she could avoid it.

Telling Mona that she "has to do it" has never worked. However, Alzheimer's has made her very docile and vulnerable when she first awakens. This is another example of learning to let the disease work for you. I can get her up from a sound sleep, dressed and ready to go in about ten minutes.

The secret is that I wake Mona up using the technique I have previously described. I have also described the variation on this pattern on Tuesdays and Thursdays when the Aide is there. The Aide is in and out and the rest of the day is free for doctor's appointments and other activities.

Avoidance and Accommodation are the only ways to deal with the real or anticipated behavior of an Alzheimer's victim. Except in the instance of immediate danger, the criteria for applying one or the other is discretionary. For example, one may Avoid situations, which are annoying, but not dangerous or Accommodate a situation for one's own benefit.

Please note that Avoidance and Accommodation are not only mutually exclusive, if one does neither, serious consequences may follow. If one does not or cannot Avoid the situation, one must Accommodate it. If one cannot Accommodate it, one must Avoid it.

The ultimate Avoidance, of course, is confining the Alzheimer's victim in a Nursing Home. The ultimate Accommodation is to allow the victim complete freedom while maintaining as high a level of surveillance of the victim as is necessary to assure health and safety. Rationality lies somewhere in between. The Carekeeper's responsibility is to find where.

Now I'd like to suggest some strategies for Avoiding or Accommodating a variety of behaviors that I have encountered with Mona. I do not offer them as hard and fast rules, but merely as how I handle things. I will bet that you can think of a better way. However, you first have to be receptive to the notion that there is a way to handle any situation.

Stop Trying To Teach

We are all teachers in the sense that when asked a question, we not only provide an answer, but we also try to make sure the questioner understands it. If we see dangerous or improper behavior, we not only correct it, but we also try to explain why we do not tolerate it. That works with two and three year olds, but not with an Alzheimer's victim.

Not only won't it work, it is a waste of vital energy. Almost anyone who knows me will agree that if you ask me a question, there is a high probability that I will tell you far more than you want or need to know. To do otherwise would take an effort on my part, which I am unwilling to make because I want you to have as complete an answer as I can provide.

When someone repeats the same question every few minutes, that effort can become exhausting and that doesn't benefit anyone. Make your response as concise as possible, not only because there is a better chance of the victim understand also because it takes less effort. Remember, "I don't know" probably will not be challenged.

Make Quick And Clear Decisions

This is particularly important, because when an Alzheimer's victim requests a decision, unlike when they ask for information, "I don't know", "I don't care" will not work. Accept the question as if it had been phrased as "Do you have an objection to …"

For example, "Do you want me to close the window?" has nothing to do with concern for you. It is more likely the result of the questioner feeling a draft or being cold, and if you say "No" or "I don't care", they are not sure what to do because they do not know if you share the perceived discomfort. On the other hand, if you say, "Yes" it validates the questioner's action. "Yes" is usually the best choice because it may close the issue, even if you are now going to be a little uncomfortable. However, there is no guarantee that the next question will not be, "Do you want me to open the window?" but at least you have a fifty-fifty chance.

You Don't Have To Do Everything

The victim wants to contribute. Learn to channel that need <u>and</u> energy to something productive, even if that activity might seem inappropriate.

They collect our trash on Wednesdays, requiring the delivery of a wheeled trash receptacle and a recycling box to the curb. In most households, that is considered men's work, even though it isn't very strenuous.

In our house, for a long time, it had been Mona's job and she does it willingly. To help her remember, I refer to the day as Trash Wednesday.

However, accepting that assignment does not mean Mona understands it. One Tuesday evening Mona went upstairs early and rather than call her back down, I rolled the large, nearly full trash barrel and the recycle box out to the curb. Then I went up to bed.

A couple hours later, Mona got up to go to the bathroom. Looking out the window, she saw the trash barrel at the end of the driveway. Something must have told her that she hadn't taken it out there. She went downstairs, put on a coat and brought it back in.

Recently, she has abandoned the task entirely and does not appear to understand what I am doing. That is another sad milestone along her difficult road.

Another example is that for forty years, Mona prepared all the meals and cleaned up after them. That is the way she wanted it. That was her time and she took a great deal of satisfaction from it. She no longer can.

Structure Your Private Time and Jealously Guard It

This is something that I readily admit I did not do often enough at first and when I did, I didn't do it very well. However, part of the problem is that I work at home and have no built in ways to escape. I am getting much better at this task.

If I have to do any major shopping, I do it early in the morning, before Mona is up. If I have to go out for something later in the day, I disguise it as a trip to the Post Office, the bank or the gas station, none of which interest Mona. Then I pick up whatever we need while I am out.

I also get up earlier on Sundays than the rest of the week. I do not turn on the TV or radio. There is just me, my coffee and the newspaper.

All of that helps my mental health.

Be Vigilant Without Being Involved

Losing things is a constant occurrence. Shoes, glasses, pocketbook, calendar, pens, it is always something and usually more than one something. Searching for things lost by an Alzheimer's patient could be a full time job, with plenty of over-time.

One must learn that if one sees a pair of glasses and knows the victim has on a pair, stick the unused pair in your pocket and as soon as you can, put it in the receptacle you have designated for such things. That will save a great deal of time.

If Mona comes to me with a sneaker in her hand and says, "I only have one sneaker", I take it from her, but I do not start to look for the other. When she comes up to me a few minutes later with a sneaker in her hand and says the same thing, I give her the one I already have and I am a hero.

The worst part of it is that since there is no logic involved in the loss, there can be no logic to the search. "Where did you have it last?" is an inoperable question.

However, that isn't as bad as when I see Mona searching for something that she hasn't told me was lost. That becomes vaudeville time. I ask, "What are you looking for?" She replies, "I don't know". I can never resist the obvious, "How will you know when you find it?" Sometimes that makes us sad.

Do not search. It will drive you crazy. If you go into the bathroom you should look around on your way and while you are in there, but do not search.

Think about it. The chances are that since it was lost, the patient has been in a limited number of places and eventually she will find it. It didn't go anywhere. She will soon forget it was lost.

If you do join the search, the chances are good that one of two things will occur. The first is that after a short time, the victim will ask what you are looking for and you will realize that you are the only one looking. The second is that after a while, you will suddenly notice that he or she is wearing the lost item, because she had found it and forgotten it was lost.

Don't Be Afraid To Let "Stuff" Happen

At least at this time, Mona wants very much to contribute to our life. I don't know what the experts have to say about that, but I think it is a good idea. However, that does not mean that I don't have to pay attention to the way she is contributing.

For example, at least early on cooking can be okay with certain reservations. You have to be watchful for a fry pan left on the heat, not only because it may catch fire but also because the handle will be hot.

Mopping floors and doing laundry also have risks, but I think in most cases, it is better to let people succeed if they can than to show or tell them that they can't. You can clean up later.

Get Really Angry Once In A While

Your reaction to the patient's behavior or idiosyncrasies is definitely dependent on your mood and it is always better to leave that out of the equation. However, we are all human and we have limits to our patience.

Most people would agree that I am a very patient, almost unflappable person, but I found early on in this experience that losing your cool could be therapeutic at times. When that happens, let it go. The patient will not cry harder at that than at a less strong reproach or even sarcasm, and he or she will not remember it. It is important, however, to note that I do not mean anything physical, here. There is never a reason or excuse for that.

However, it is important get over that anger. Walk it off for a few minutes. Then come back, changing the subject, preferably with some humor. Do not feel guilty. That won't help either of you. Get it out and go on.

CHAPTER 9

▼

FROM CRUISE CONTROL TO A RHYTHM OF LIFE

This chapter is the corollary to Chapter Three about putting on your oxygen mask before caring for the children. This time I will talk about ways that I have found to convert that admonition into the manner in which *I* began to live *our* life. Once again the details of how I approached this task are just that and therefore not necessarily applicable to another person's situation. I believe however, that the underlying principles are valid and should help you to find your own way.

In the previous chapter, I mentioned the desirability of determining one's cruising speed and then engaging cruise control. Although I had intended to develop that analogy in this chapter as I began this paragraph the title of a song from the 1969 Broadway musical "Sweet Charity" flashed into my mind. The song is "The Rhythm of Life" and although the lyrics are not applicable, the title conveys the concept I was trying to describe much better than "cruising speed".

The role of a Carekeeper for an Alzheimer's victim, as with victims of many other diseases, is a 24/7/365 proposition and often one really has no idea what will happen next. In some ways, it is a tightly scheduled almost frantic existence but not in all. "Cruising speed" implies a constant rate of activity. Developing a rhythm of life is a much more apt description of the objective.

Different situations require changes in tempo, the intensity of the beat, both or neither and the trick is to understand which, is the appropriate response. Sometimes issues arise with the victim that demand the tempo increase but at other times, slowing the tempo is more appropriate. More often than one might expect, it is just better to go with the flow. Not all reactions are time sensitive and you will see that sometimes it is easier and more effective to let the situation play out and make the necessary repairs after the fact, rather than to intervene. The objective however, is to establish a consistent basic rhythm, to which one can return.

I know virtually nothing about opera although I usually listen to it on Saturday afternoons as background music while I work on the computer. If I have been told the story I can usually (although not always) follow the action even when it is in an unfamiliar language. That is because the rhythm of the life in which the characters exist reflects developments in the story. I sometimes think that when I lose track of the action at least part of the blame belongs to the composer, who lost his rhythm.

One cannot reach a rhythm of life all at once. After several years, mine is still a work in process replete with frustrations. Nonetheless, it is constantly albeit slowly becoming more serene. I made very little progress until I discovered yet another counter-intuitive reality. I had been trying to develop a rhythm of our life. That will never work. There is no rhythm to the life of an Alzheimer's victim. On the other hand, perhaps there are too many, completely random and in conflict.

One cannot plan and manage chaos, but merely prepare to accommodate it. Although the structured portion of Mona's life is an element of that rhythm, her behavior has increasingly become an interruption. My lifestyle provides the underlying rhythm for both of us. That way, I could deal with the necessary and unpredictable changes in tempo or intensity and sometimes both, yet ultimately return smoothly to the underlying rhythm.

The game of golf can teach us many lessons. One, which applies here, is the way the great players maintain their routine under all circumstances. Whether they are playing well or poorly often is imperceptible to the casual observer. If distracted when about to take a shot, they do not react, but back away and start over from the beginning, as if they planned it that way. They re-mark the ball and line up the putt again on the green, re-tee the ball on the tee, or act as if they had just walked up to the ball and discovered it in the fairway, rough or bunker.

Using these rituals allows them to re-establish their personal rhythm and reduce, if not eliminate distractions and emotion. Although each is doing the same thing, they have found their own on-course rhythm of life. If one looks closely, the difference between Tiger Woods and Sergio Garcia is obvious, but each has a rhythm, setting them apart from their less successful peers.

In contrast, the emotions of the not-so-great players are transparent. When I was working with them regularly, I could walk onto a golf course during an LPGA tournament and without looking at a leader board, know how some golfers were playing by the speed they walked, the way they held their heads or the way they swung their arms. One LPGA player, who I know very well and consider a good friend always swung her arms straight forward and back when she was at par or better and across her body when she was not. Unfortunately, that pattern could and would change after one bad shot.

One Sunday the last day of the tournament, she was leading by two shots. I walked with her from the practice area to the first tee and was pleased to note that she was swinging her arms in the right direction.

She hit her first shot fairly well, but it was a little short and not in perfect position. She turned toward me and said, "See, I told you I couldn't play this game". Off she went down the fairway, arms swinging side to side. She finished third.

Developing a workable rhythm of life for the care of an Alzheimer's victim requires four steps:

- Establish the Carekeeper's rhythm of life without reference to that of the victim.

- Apply the Administrative and Maintenance elements of the victim's life to that rhythm to establish the household rhythm of life.

- Establish and schedule the Carekeeper's private time and the related activities within the context of the basic rhythm.

- Learn to deal with disruptions.

We will look at the first two of these in this chapter and the other two in the next. I will first describe the rhythm of my life for a typical week, without any reference to Mona. Then I will super-impose Mona's Administrative and Maintenance requirements.

Establishing The Carekeeper's Rhythm Of Life

This section covers what I have done, as well as some things I plan to do but have not yet integrated. I am certain that some of these will not suit everyone. In fact, I can't imagine all would completely suit anyone but me and perhaps others would suit me even better. Each person must establish his or her unique rhythm of life.

Doing this involved a major change in my lifestyle and perhaps in my personality. I had to learn to be responsive, not just reactive. I had to learn that fire protection is far more efficient than fire fighting and repairing or cleaning up may be less stressful than intervention. Most of all, I had to become far less judgmental than I have ever been.

I also had to learn that in order to work properly, one's rhythm of life must be interesting and diverse. If it is not, one can be lulled into inattention. To do that I had to learn that relaxing does not necessarily mean taking a nap, although sometimes that is also a good idea. On the other hand, some people fight bulls or skydive for relaxation.

This effort requires two equally important things:

- Possess the willingness, capability and determination to explicitly factor frequent and sizable blocks of time into your life for your personal use.

- Use imagination to develop interesting, challenging and worthwhile activities to fill that time.

Just having the first will bore you to death. If you just have the second, your problem will be massive frustration for two reasons: you know that those activities are good for you and outside factors are preventing you from doing them. You must remember that you have only yourself to blame. That situation is not the victim's fault.

The bottom line is that Carekeepers must be the composers and stars of their own live operas. They must establish the rhythm of their lives, even though the demands of the victim influence its structure.

The first two conditions I set were that I need sufficient sleep to remain fully functional and I should always start and end each day in a reasonable state of serenity. To those initial guidelines, I added the desirability of returning to that serene state at least once during the day.

I believe it is essential for one to have a regular self-imposed routine and timetable, built around immutable things especially if one is over the age of sixty. Therefore, I established 7:30 AM as my wake up time and 11:30 PM as my bedtime. The normal tolerance on each is half an hour.

This was a major departure from my life up to that point. For many years prior, I would always start with the latest time at which I could begin my first task of the day and then work back using minimum times for getting ready, but without factoring any contingency time to the moment I had to leap out of bed. The result was that my morning rhythm was staccato and often out of control. Now I settle into my rhythm gradually and get to my first task right on the beat.

At the other end of the day, I usually resisted going to sleep until that option became more interesting than what I was doing. That often made for short nights. Changing that took discipline and persistence.

I have an alarm set for my "fail safe" time to awake, but it rarely sounds. I spend my first few minutes in prayer in bed, to establish serenity and set my rhythm. Then I rise, brush my teeth, shave, shower leisurely and get dressed. My pace is unhurried but deliberate as it reaches its desired rhythm.

Because Mona is easiest to handle when she is waking up, I try to arrange that she awake not on my schedule, but on one that I established for her. To avoid waking her prematurely, I keep my clothes in my office closet and I use the main bathroom, rather than the one off our bedroom.

I have a strong interest in a very broad spectrum of current events and I feel it is important for me to keep in touch with the world outside our home. Therefore, as soon as I have shaved, showered and dressed, I sit at my computer, where I read any overnight e-mail, scan the on-line versions of the New York Times as well as the Rochester and Syracuse newspapers, check out a favorite golf Forum and read the latest world headlines on Google News.

Moving downstairs, I turn on CNN, retrieve the newspaper, put my morning oatmeal in the microwave and let the dog out. Before the oatmeal is ready, I have a pot of coffee brewing.

When I finish my breakfast, I clean up the dishes, fill a thermos carafe with coffee and head back upstairs to my office and the computer. I am still on rhythm and still serene.

I am the Moderator of two medium sized Internet Forums, and although that does not entail very much work, I always check them to make sure there are no problems. Then I log onto a classical music website to start the background music for my day. Usually, Mona's wake up time has not yet arrived.

I review the day's tasks, making adjustments as required. As a Carekeeper, I have many demands on my time. Factoring sizable blocks of it into my life requires rigorous time management. There are many systems for doing that on the market, but I use a computer program called Microsoft Outlook. It handles my e-mail, my calendar and my Task List, all the necessary elements of time management. If something does not appear in Outlook, I may not do it. Stated more accurately, I enter everything that I need to do in Outlook and then maintain it meticulously.

However, for a Carekeeper to be successful at managing his or her time also requires that one become what others consider somewhat counter-intuitive in the establishment of priorities. The top priority, of course, must be maintaining the health and safety of the victim in your care, but a close second is maintaining the rigor of assuring those sizable blocks of private time. Do not confuse this with slack time, which is a buffer to handle unanticipated delays. Private time is just that and should always be planned so that it is not squandered.

The competition for that personal time must be of equal or greater priority than all the routine things in your and the victim's lives. Anything else you must do ranks last.

You must learn to schedule those Carekeeper related elements, including the victim's medical appointments around your private time without shortchanging yourself. The sooner you develop that habit, the better. As for many things, the secret is discipline although this is a very personal process. I can only tell you what I have done. I hope you will be able to follow the pattern.

I have two kinds of time available during which I can schedule personal activities. The first is that when Mona is essentially in the custody of someone else. Usually, that means between 10:00 AM and 4:30 PM on Mondays, Wednesdays and Fridays when she is at Day Care and for an hour each on Tuesdays and Thursdays when the Aide is here.

When Mona first began to go to Day Care, both friends and family expressed pleasure that I was going to have three more or less full days "to do whatever you want". There is that need for counter-intuitive thinking again. I must spend part of that time doing the things I must do for us that I cannot do at home. I have to work that in around my blocks of personal time.

I personally like to get the routine stuff out of the way, so I try to do it first. That does not mean I give it higher priority. If I do not have enough time in one day to accommodate that personal time, I make up the personal time on another day. Treat it as a zero sum game. For example, if I plan on six hours of personal time outside of the house for the week it doesn't have to be two hours per day, but it must be six hours during each week.

Establish priorities because there are a number of routine tasks to do outside the house and you cannot do them efficiently with the victim in tow. They include the laundry, shopping, personal and pet appointments, banking, doctors' visits, haircuts, getting the car serviced and business appointments. These are personal tasks although they do not qualify under the definition of personal time used here. Those are administrative and maintenance tasks and that is an important distinction.

These things can eat up a lot of Mondays, Wednesdays and Fridays. Despite that, you must earmark some of that time away from the house for private time, preferably out of doors when the weather permits.

In order to balance one's priorities effectively, some strong, hierarchical guidelines and creative planning are required to optimize your rhythm of life. In turn, they can also provide the opportunity for refreshing and interesting personal time. My own guidelines are certainly strong, hierarchical and simple:

- Never blow an entire day on administrative and maintenance tasks.

- Don't let chores like doing laundry or having the car serviced become spectator sports.

- Never return home without accomplishing at least two things.

- Never pass up the opportunity to do something unexpected and interesting.

In theory, one could probably compress all the tasks for the week into one or two days, but that could take far more effort than it is worth. However, spreading them evenly across the three days can preclude you from ever feeling that you are really "playing hooky" and that is not good.

Doing laundry on a timely basis is essential. However, as I said earlier, with a little investment and some experimentation, I have reached the point where I need to do it no more often than every thirteen days. I operate on a three-week cycle of Monday the first week, Friday the second and not at all in the third.

I generally try to schedule other administrative and maintenance appointments, except for grocery shopping so that they do not occur on laundry days, although sometimes that is not possible. By having all the dirty clothes in laundry bags before Mona gets up, all I have to do is strip our bed while she is in the bathroom and I am ready to leave as soon as she is picked up for Day Care.

The laundry takes approximately two and a half hours, door to door. However, there is about forty minutes of potential spectator time during the wash cycle and over an hour more while the dryers are running. To conform to my second guideline I drink my morning coffee, eat a breakfast croissant and read the newspaper during the wash cycle.

I satisfy that same guideline by making a trip to the grocery store during the drying cycle. I rarely buy anything at a store without knowing exactly when and how I am going to use it, so this is not recreational shopping. With that constraint, I can buy at least $90 worth of groceries and be back before the dryers stop. That also takes care of my third guideline, as well as my first, because I still have most of the afternoon free.

Obviously, you must schedule other obligatory activities and miscellaneous errands. To the fullest extent possible, I try to schedule them so that all together they occupy no more than half of one of the non-laundry days. Once again I observe my four guidelines: never blow an entire day, don't let chores become a spectator sport, never return home without accomplishing at least two things, and especially, do not pass up something unexpected and interesting. That way, I always have at least one full day to myself each week and every third week I have two.

Applying the Victim's Requirements To Establish The Household Rhythm Of Life

There are some unique things pertinent for those Carekeepers who are the spouses or children of the victim. Alzheimer's Disease makes many changes in relationships, but few as profound as those between close and intimate relatives do. The Carekeeper must accept those changes without guilt in order to do his or her job and maintain their own well-being. One must learn to live in the reality of the present. After all, that is the only place the victim really is.

For over fifty years, most of the decisions I made were in the context of Mona's preferences, likes and dislikes, comfort and feelings. As a result, usually the de facto final decision among alternatives was hers. That is not only no longer necessary it is no longer possible. The Alzheimer's victims reach a point when they do not remember preferences, likes and dislikes and don't know what makes them comfortable or feel better.

That is not to say that they are unhappy, just that they are content to have direction. As I mentioned earlier, I have found that this extends to food preferences, which may sound insignificant, but really is not.

In terms of establishing the rhythm of your household, this provides you with considerable freedom in dealing with the victim's administrative/maintenance needs so that they do not impinge on your personal/therapeutic activities. The important distinction is that because the victim is not in charge, the Carekeeper must be.

I must admit that occasionally in frustration, I remind Mona of this new relationship and that she is no longer in charge. That is a very bad practice and I must avoid it because it is gratuitous, hurtful and has no effect. It also makes you both feel bad and ironically, the Carekeeper feels bad about it for a much longer time.

My scheduling challenge is mostly limited to Tuesdays and Thursdays when Mona is not at Day Care. On those days, the Home Health Care Aide visits to check on Mona's general condition and to assist her in her personal hygiene needs. She arrives at 8:15 AM, so Mona is up early.

In addition, every other Tuesday a Visiting Nurse stops by for about half an hour to give Mona a cursory medical check and talk with me about changes in medications, behavior, attitude or anything else I have noticed. Since the Visiting Nurse is also there to check on the work of the Aide, usually the visits overlap to some degree. In any case, half of the Tuesday visits are over by ten and all of the Thursday visits are over by nine-fifteen.

Getting Mona up and off somewhere is easiest to manage with a sense of controlled urgency, keeping her constantly moving without much time to reflect. It is like an interval of ragtime, returning to the basic rhythm of life when she is finally in the car.

Therefore, insofar as possible, appointments with Mona's doctor and other activities requiring her physical presence I schedule for mid-morning. After that, Mona is free to do pretty much whatever she wants, within the limits of health and safety.

Weekends are a very different situation. On Saturdays, I let Mona determine when she gets up and that is rarely before one or two in the afternoon. Obviously, that gives me freedom for a good part of the day. Mona sleeps so soundly and with so little chance of her getting up that, I am confident in leaving for as much as two hours in the morning.

I let Mona sleep late on Sunday as well, not waking her until it is time to go to church. It is also a different kind of day for me as well, because we spend most of it in each other's company.

These things make up the Rhythm of Our Life and please note that I did not say lives.

In the next chapter, I will discuss choosing the Carekeepers' activities that will occupy those blocks of private time as well as how to minimize and deal with disruptions by the victim. There is no science in that, but a great deal of art.

CHAPTER 10

▼

ENJOYING PRIVATE TIME
AND DEALING WITH
DISRUPTION

It would be difficult for me to overemphasize the importance to the Carekeeper of establishing and managing his or her private time. It is the difference between freedom and a form of imprisonment. It is a non-chemical defense against depression. It is the difference between remaining whole and shriveling beyond recognition.

It is really a dress rehearsal for the rest of one's life. Do not take it lightly.

Remember that establishing and managing one's private time can only be done against the backdrop of the common underlying rhythm of life of the Carekeeper and the victim. Their individual rhythms are not relevant.

Although I have an established rhythm of life, Mona's life is arrhythmic. It verges on chaotic. Dealing with that has both an offensive and defensive component, depending on the activity and the behavior. The key is that the more planning one does the more one can maintain a comfortable rhythm of life and that in turn makes it easier to respond to real surprises and emergencies. This is an art, not a science.

Moreover, it is completely possible for a Carekeeper to set aside meaningful periods of personal time, which is essential to his or her mental and emotional well-being. All that it takes is desire and discipline to make it happen. The alternative is to indeed, squander a portion of one's life, perhaps at an age when one hasn't all that much left.

I suggest the following guidelines for selecting activities for your valuable private time:

- Never allow a chore to become a private time activity. Cutting the grass is a chore, but creating a garden can be a legitimate private time activity.

- Do not even fleetingly consider inherently stressful activities.

- Stay away from activities with long learning curves, unless learning and not doing is your objective.

- Consider the "interruptability factor" in evaluating an activity. Interruptions happen and if it takes considerable time to return to where you were, that can be doubly frustrating.

- Select as your primary activity, something to which you will look forward to doing even more than you look forward to the concept of having private time.

- Set levels for success, which are consistent with your enjoyment of the activity.

- Select one or more secondary and alternative activities for those times when you want or need a break from your primary private time activity.

- Have a reasonable and interesting mix of things that you do at home and of those that must or at least can do somewhere else.

- When possible select those activities, which can be enjoyed elsewhere when you have the opportunity, especially when the weather is favorable.

- Don't hesitate to drop an activity when it no longer meets your needs, but don't do that until you have a replacement. Your annoyance with the old will inspire your search for the new.

- Be on the alert for new activities, but be aware of your available time and other limitations.

Once you have fully grasped the importance of these guidelines, you are ready to manage your private time and select your primary, as well as secondary, private time activities.

Managing, Rather Than Micromanaging Your Private Time

There is a great deal of uncertainty in the day-to-day life of the Carekeeper, which makes managing private time more of an art than a science. Micromanaging by definition cannot ever become an art. This is illustrated by an example.

On the days Mona attends Day Care I have free time from about 10:00 AM to 4:30 PM, which is available for private activity. However, part of Carekeeping involves chores such as grocery shopping, laundry and meal preparation among others. It is often difficult to estimate how long those things will take.

Here is my way:

My approach is to make a game out of it. I make my private time the reward for finishing the chores in a timely fashion. That way, spending too much time on chores becomes a self-correcting problem. If it happens only rarely, I forgive myself. If not, I do something about it.

Selecting The Carekeeper's Primary Home-Based Private Time Activity

The biggest waste of time a Carekeeper can experience is in wondering rather than deciding what to do with his or her private time. However, this is not just a "make a list and pick one" exercise. The selection should be the result of the careful and deliberate consideration of alternatives based on serious criteria. The actual choice will then become obvious.

In general, your choice should be from among things that are intellectually stimulating since for the most part dealing with a person with Alzheimer's certainly is not. I would also encourage that your choice be something that does not require a great deal of set up time and that you are able to leave without having to put everything away.

There should be some variety in what you do so that your personal time does not become onerous, and in this connection, one should not be afraid to try something new. On the other hand, it would not seem wise to select an activity, which requires a long learning curve. That can become very frustrating and frustration is what you are trying to avoid.

It is good for these activities to have physical as well as mental components as long as they are within your capabilities. You need neither injury nor exhaustion. Most important of all is that one's private time activities should be fun in the sense that they are things to which you look forward. You already have enough drudgery in your life to run a major sale on e-Bay.

Finally, you must establish a specific place in which to spend your personal time, preferably one where there is some degree of privacy. However, one should avoid allowing that place to become a personal prison. I also found it wise to make it clear from the outset that when Mona entered that place, my office she was a guest on my turf and not expected to dawdle.

Therefore, it seemed logical to me that one's primary private time activity should meet rather strict criteria, which included:

- If possible, it should be something that you have always wanted to do "if I just had the time". Believe me it doesn't get any better than that, since it is its own reward.

- It should be weatherproof, which in our climate means that it is primarily an indoor activity and something that will capture and hold one's interest sufficiently that you don't care if it is not possible to leave the house. However, if you are either very creative or very fortunate, it may have a viable outside or at least away from home component. Mine does.

- It should be long term in nature at least in terms of the talents, skills and equipment used. In other words, a series of related or unrelated projects employing the same skill set is acceptable, perhaps even preferable. This describes my personal choice of writing.

- The activity should have its own defined place where access can be limited and where you keep the tools and the work in process. Limiting the access of the Alzheimer's victim is particularly important. However, this does not mean that you can be so isolated that you cannot be aware of the person whose care you are keeping. For me, that place is my office.

- The activity should be interruptible in the sense that you can stop it almost immediately and re-start without great effort. Avoid things like cutting diamonds.

- Typically, such activities are sedentary pursuits, but that is not a necessity. For example, exercise and fitness activities could fit this definition.

Here is my way:

There is a current commercial running on TV and as is often the case I don't remember the sponsor but it has a message that is more relevant than any product. The scene is a custom automobile shop and the grizzled owner is telling a client that he has sold the business. He explains, "I just decided that I had to chase a dream before I'm too old to do it".

The next scene is the arrival of the new owner, apparently a successful executive. By way of introducing himself while displaying both his interest and skill by his body language he says, "I just decided that I had to chase a dream before I'm too old to do it".

This can be an opportunity to fulfill your own dream. If you can, indulge yourself by doing something you always wanted to do. Make that a tribute to your devotion as a Carekeeper, not just something to keep you occupied or entertained.

From the time I was a junior in high school, I have wanted to be a writer. At that early age and through college and graduate school, I wrote turgid and pretentious prose, nearly all fiction, and accumulated stacks of rejection letters. In the fifty years since, in connection with my work I have no doubt written enough reports, letters, plans and proposals to fill several walls of bookshelves, but little of it has been the kind of writing that I really wanted to do.

Several years before Mona's diagnosis of Alzheimer's, I seriously began to write things for myself again. I became determined that as soon as I could, I would write full time.

My children and theirs prompted my first attempt, a collection of stories I have been telling for years. They are mostly about funny things that either happened to me or that I have done. I have grouped them by decades and "Decades" is the title of the book. I am about in the middle of the nineteen fifties.

Although they were not limited to Mona's illness, a series of things had put a strain on my personal faith and distracted me from that project. I found that writing about that personal struggle helped me to handle it. The result was a book called "The Compliant, Curious & Critical Catholic: Three Ordinary Persons In One Guy". I have finished and published the book and I feel very good about that, but most amazing was its therapeutic effect.

There was no hesitation on my part in the selection of writing as my "Primary Private Time" activity and I will not bore you by gushing over the reasons why it is right for me, except to say that it was not so that I could write _this_ book. That would have been an exercise in wallowing and perhaps self-pity. I hope it didn't turn out that way.

Therefore, it is ironic that while dealing with Mona's Alzheimer's Disease I found the subject matter for this second book. I am pleased that this was not my first and I am certain it won't be my last. However, I strongly believe and devoutly hope this will be the only one I will ever write on this subject.

My first one was very different and my next one, already started is just as different from the first two. All the others I have planned will be different. At my age, I don't have time to do the same thing twice. I hope I get to some fiction. I think my turgidity is either cured or at least in remission.

The cornerstone of the activities I do for myself is writing. I can truthfully say that I have yet to experience sitting staring at a blank computer screen with no idea of how to begin. I try to write for several hours a day, mostly against a background of classical music and I usually succeed. I have not, however learned very much about classical music.

Selecting The Carekeeper's Alternate Home Based Private Time Activities

Regardless of how much one enjoys an activity, there are times when you just want to do something else. In selecting alternate private time activities, the Carekeeper might consider these additional criteria:

- Ideally, they should employ a different skill set. For example, if one's primary activity is computer based, a great alternative might be playing a musical instrument. However, if one hadn't thought of it years ago, that may not be very practical.

- If it employs the same skill set, its content should be different enough to make the experience seem different.

In other words, make it a real alternative.

Here is my way:

I realize that my approach to this challenge may appear to contradict some of the things I have just said. Just remember that my program is a work in progress and not perfect. Once again, it is not a formula but an approach. You may well have a better one.

I said earlier that the only difficulty with choosing one activity is the danger of becoming bored with it. Variety is highly desirable. I have found that for me, at least a partial answer is in similar though unrelated activities. In my case, although I am not a highly technically oriented person they are mostly things that involve the use of my computer.

I maintain an extensive e-mail correspondence with friends and family. This keeps me in touch with people who, although they are keenly interested in Mona's condition really want to talk about a number of things other than that for which I am grateful. I usually allow them to interrupt whatever I am doing and people kid me about my quick responses. It helps to keep me alert.

One friend, rediscovered by e-mail after fifty years, has urged the use of "snail mail" for us to maintain contact and I am enjoying using that medium again. In many ways, it is more satisfying than the immediate, but less reflective e-mail. I have tried with modest success to do the same with my grandchildren, but that is also a work in progress.

The computer also plays a role in a third activity. As I mentioned earlier, I moderate two private, password protected, Internet Forums. One is for the Le Moyne College classes of my general era. In addition to the small amount of administrative work required, I actively try to attract new members and to stimulate discussion among those we have. Some of these people have become part of my e-mail community as well.

The other Forum is one that I set up to help an Internet-challenged friend. Initially, that occupied a great deal of my time, but recently I have become just one of many participants.

The Internet also plays a major role in my quest for information about Alzheimer's, in support of my writing and as my way to satisfy my curiosity about a number of things important and trivial, through extensive use of Google. I am also an unabashed news and political junkie, sometimes on the Internet, checking Google News and various other sources several times a day.

Selecting The Carekeeper's Away From Home Private Time Activities

Almost by definition, away from home activities can only be primary by extension and I will be discuss that aspect later. Obviously, I am referring to activities enjoyed when the victim is under someone else's care. The keyword in that sentence is "enjoyed".

There is no inherent need for commonality here. In fact, diversification is often refreshing and don't be afraid to do something frivolous or totally out of character. I have a friend, who on his fiftieth birthday, made a list of one hundred things he wanted to do before he died. They ranged from very simple to quite complex. When he turned seventy, I asked him how he was doing on his list and he said he had accomplished far more than he thought he would. Consider that approach.

This concept has its own criteria for selection:

- Concentrate on things nearby at first remembering that getting there and back takes time.

- Consider things that complement your at-home activities, such as research projects.

- Consider the obvious. There is a great deal going on around you.

- Carefully consider volunteering, making sure that it is something upbeat and happy.

- Remember that you don't always have to do something spectacular. Ordinary things newly discovered are enjoyable and worthwhile.

Within that construct, pick the total number of different things that you think you could do in the next month. Then triple that number to establish the goal for the items you put on your list. Now let your mind wander.

Here is my way:

If you are as I am, you will choose ten or fifteen items quickly and then run out of ideas. If that happens, go back over the list and let your current choices suggest others. Keep going until you have at least one third of the goal for the list.

Then copy the list neatly, but don't prioritize it. Make those decisions spontaneously. When you do something on the list, cross it out, but discipline yourself to add two for each one you complete in order to build up a backlog.

Let your imagination guide you. For example, return from your experience by a route that is different from the way you went there. Try to find ideas for other days while going there, during the time you are there and on the way home. Look for things that you can enjoy in connection with something else on your list. Don't do anything that seems like a chore and if it really is a chore drop it from the list, but remember that two items must replace each one that comes off the list.

At first, I did not do very well using those blocks of personal time for things away from home and I still am not fully functioning in this mode. As with everything, one must schedule activities. However when one lives in a climate such as I do, there must always be an alternative if the weather is inclement. Sometimes, administrative and maintenance tasks can be combined into multi-purpose trips and scheduled around a visit to a park or a museum.

Be creative in your approach and don't forget the things that are right under your nose. Most cities of any size have things, which can provide the interest and all the necessary simple pleasure but you overlook them. When I was in graduate school at Fordham I lived in New York City for a year, but I never visited the Statue of Liberty. We lived in Washington, DC for three years and I never went into the Washington Monument. I still have done neither.

I have lived in the Rochester, NY area for over forty years and I quickly made a list of twenty or more things that I have not done or seen and would like to. It just takes a little thinking about it.

When you have an appointment, try to visualize two or three alternate routes to or from your destination. Then visualize the things that you will pass along each alternative route. The chances are that you will come up with something that doesn't take much time and that you have not done in a long time or maybe even ever. Then do it. Each time it will be easier and more enjoyable.

There is a strong temptation when your principal, private diversion is an indoor activity like writing to stay home and work on that, especially if you *really* enjoy it. Save that for days when the weather is bad and try to spend at least half of every available good day outside doing something that is not administration or maintenance.

Your diversion doesn't have to be a place. It can be food. Sometimes it can be both. Last summer, ferry service began from Rochester across Lake Ontario to Toronto. The ferry is a large, twin hulled craft carrying 750 passengers and about 400 cars. I had never seen it.

One day I saw that an excellent Japanese restaurant in the area had opened a new Sushi Bar in the Ferry Terminal, which is located in a park at the mouth of the Genesee River. Mona does not particularly like sushi, so one beautiful summer day as soon as she left for Day Care I made the half hour drive to the lake.

I watched the ferry pull out and head for Toronto, walked a couple of miles on the beach and finished my morning with a lunch of delicious sushi, accompanied by a bottle of Kirin Beer. I felt like I had been on a vacation.

I must admit that I have not had many days like that one, but I am determined to change that situation. As the weather worsens, I have a list of indoor places to visit. In addition, the golf foursome with whom I played for thirty-five years has established a regular monthly lunch together.

Some elements are sorely missing from my current activities. They are those that are physical in nature and those that involve very new experiences. Outside activities have had less priority than they should and I am going to work on that. As a former avid golfer, I have always spent a great deal of time outside in the seven months we can do that in western New York. Since my business was producing corporate golf outings, golf courses and the out of doors often were my office year round.

Golf became less of an option a few years ago when I suffered a rotator cuff injury, which is not repairable. The result is that I curtailed my outside activities greatly in the past few years albeit more from neglect than design, but I am determined to change that. In nearly every direction from our house, one encounters at least one large park within a very few miles. I am promising myself lunch in the park at least once per week as soon as the weather improves.

In the meantime, I need to get on with the visits to local places where I have never been or at least have not seen in years. I also need to get on with my informal education.

Selecting And Scheduling The Carekeeper's Semi-Private Time Activities

Companionship is important in Carekeeping and you should have some Semi-Private Time activities, which you enjoy in the presence even if not with the participation of the Alzheimer's victim. These should be included in your private time program.

Perhaps program is not the appropriate word here. This is really just living the shared life you have with the person in your care. It is just as mundane as the lives of anyone else. The difference is that in these activities, you can count on interruptions.

I feel that this semi-private time is an important part of maintaining Mona's life as close to normal as possible. That is the way we have lived it for more than fifty years. It is also a defense against having to watch Mona's constant COD behavior.

The semi-private activity consists of a combination of three or four elements: reading the morning paper, which I hide all day so I am sure I have it; preparing and eating meals; watching selected TV programming; or watching DVD movies.

For one's own sanity, a DVR on the TV is essential so that programs can be paused or run backwards after the inevitable interruptions. My advice is to sign up for DVR service from your cable provider if it is available and make hitting the pause button an automatic response. That will lower your blood pressure, relieve your stress and probably extend your life.

This version of semi-private time is inherently vulnerable to frequent interruption and you must plan for that.

When Mona is in my care at home, normally Tuesdays, Thursdays, Saturdays and Sundays, she is on her own during the day although I am just a step away. She is free to fix whatever she wants to eat during the day, but if she hasn't had lunch by one o'clock, I fix something for her. In that regard, it is important to have things available to fix.

Here is my way:

At around six, I join Mona for dinner and the evening, but that does not mean I haven't seen her all day. I check on her regularly.

I rarely pursue my non-computer personal activities such as reading in the office because that does not represent a change of routine and I refuse to watch videos on my computer. I watch TV or read in the family room, or do the latter on the back porch in good weather. Often Mona is present when I am doing these things and in a sense, it appears that we are doing them together. However, it would be more accurate to say that we are doing them separately and simultaneously in the same place, since Mona is at the point when she doesn't really participate in such things.

I do continue my pursuit of news and politics off the computer, sometimes with TV and always through the newspaper. Having said that, I try to limit my TV news intake, tuning out as soon as it becomes repetitious or partisan which is often.

I am quite selective in my other TV viewing, limiting it to six or eight hours per week, mostly dramas each at least an hour in length with the quality of the writing being my main criteria. I watch football and golf and Mona enjoys both of them. I do not watch sitcoms. I do turn the TV off when there is nothing that meets <u>my</u> criteria. I try to read, but often find that my attention span is short and when Mona is present, interruptions are frequent.

Strangely, I do some of my personal activity in the kitchen. Mona was a dedicated and excellent chef and I had serious misgivings when I realized that I had to assume those duties. In addition, I didn't think I really wanted to cook.

However, I soon discovered that Mona had taught me a great deal and I think I have some natural talent. At least I am not afraid to fail and in some ways, I think I am much more creative than Mona is, often straying from the recipe if I even follow one, to experiment.

My repertoire is still rather limited and I'm big on the use of a crockpot. However, I have a rule to cook nothing in the crockpot that includes the contents of more than one can. Somehow, I feel dumping more than one can into a crockpot is making it too easy and less creative. I work at that and I enjoy doing it.

Learning to Deal With Disruptions

Now, remembering that the objective is to allow *me* to return to and maintain *my* rhythm of life let's look at how Mona's behavior impinges on it. Note that I did not say behavior patterns, because the nature of an Alzheimer's victim even in the Moderate stage is patternless.

Obviously, the inherent arrhythmia of Mona's life and the effects of her behavior affect me only during those times when she is under my supervision.

Ironically, there are many opportunities for personal time on the days when Mona is at home all day. That is not to say, however, that those are times without interruption. Therefore, one should select personal activities for those days that can accommodate distraction, lest the aggravation be greater than the pleasure. Furthermore, one should *expect* interruption.

As I said, I never watch television or read the newspaper in my office, even though that dramatically increases my vulnerability to interruption or its sibling, distraction. Those things are inevitable and one must develop coping strategies.

There are two basic types of disruptive behavior: those occurring *independently* of what I am doing and those occurring *because* of what I am doing. The former can and do occur at anytime, but they only affect the rhythm of our life when I allow myself to be aware of them.

Examples of things, which occur independently, are standing in front of the TV set, re-arranging things on the shelves while I am watching a program and disrupting with trivial things, including putting on strange hats when I am reading or talking on the telephone. They also include asking me to come and see things outside, in the other room or upstairs while I am trying to prepare dinner. Mona is, in effect, oblivious to what I am doing.

Most of the things she does *because* of what I am doing have to do with the preparation of food, which I suspect is an expression of her wanting to help. They include washing and putting away utensils I am using and have set down for a moment and putting away ingredients I have set out to use, usually putting them in bizarre places. They also include generally being in the way of me doing things and changing the temperature of things cooking at medium to high heat, low or even off when I am not looking.

These latter things can be counter-productive, overly disruptive and usually produce more stress in me. I try constantly to develop strategies to combat these behaviors, which further tends to exacerbate their effect on me.

Here is my way:

My preferred defense regarding disruptive behaviors occurring *independently* of what I am doing is to ignore them, although that judgment always involves consideration of whether the activity is dangerous or not. For example if her rearranging involves standing on a chair to reach the top shelf, I will offer to help.

When the disruptive behaviors are *because* of what I am doing, I react quickly and decisively, because they might sabotage my efforts. I will however, admit that I discovered early on that when I took that kind of action, Mona's reaction often appeared to be annoyance that I was rejecting her expert assistance. She apparently decided that I was not worthy of help and she stopped offering it. Sometimes I must elevate my dudgeon to get that response, but when I do she retreats and pouts. Pouting I can handle.

CHAPTER 11

▼

ACCEPTING THE PRESENT AND PLANNING FOR THE FUTURE

For a number of reasons this is the most difficult chapter for me to write and I suspect that it will be difficult for many to read. In a sense, I am going to outline the conditions under which I will have failed at what I set out to do. Some may interpret that as saying, "Yes, I love Mona and I will continue to *help* care for her, but ..."

To some extent that is accurate since clearly someone perhaps stronger or better qualified than I will take over Mona's care at some point. That certainly does not mean that I will abandon her. It just means that she and I will have moved into another phase of the battle with Alzheimer's Disease, which we cannot win. It is likely this step will be one she hardly notices and I will grieve.

This also means that I have completed my work with Mona. I am determined that when that happens, I will be proud of what I accomplished, and I will not be concerned if others attempt to second guess.

In an earlier chapter, I mentioned that the most severe loss I suffered when Mona contracted Alzheimer's was a loss of intimacy. By that, I meant the constant interaction of two people sharing one life, making decisions large and small without concern about whether they affect the other because they were joint decisions. It is the confidence that when a decision is about to be made, a look, a smile, a shrug or a touch can affirm or modify it, without a word spoken. Yet when the time comes to make *this* decision, no matter how hard I look, I will see no signal.

I have shared more than seventy-five percent of Mona's life experiences, yet only I remember them. One night a couple of weeks ago, she shook me to wake me up. When I was awake, she asked gently "Who are you?" I told her and her response was, "Oh, that's good. That is what I thought, but I wanted to be sure".

That exchange was not as heartbreaking as it may sound. For her it was comforting, not traumatic. I understood it was part of the experience just the inevitability of Alzheimer's Disease and I made peace with that long ago. It validated that my fifty-two year investment had earned enough trust to be verifiable by a confused mind operating in total darkness. Therefore, in a way, it was comforting for me as well.

Nonetheless, from the beginning, I have known that ultimately this is a decision I will have to make and I am the one who can.

Long before I began this book, I saw an article in the newspaper about a man who lives nearby and who recently was diagnosed with early onset Alzheimer's. The article dealt with the way in which he and his wife were handling the situation.

I sent his wife a note enclosing the fourteen-page piece I had written about Mona for our friends and family before our granddaughter Shannon's wedding in 2003. Two days later, I had a call not from her, but her husband.

He thanked me and told me in some detail how they were dealing with his diagnosis. This was a surprising turn of events, but I realized that he had been diagnosed very early no doubt because he has the genetic form of Alzheimer's Disease, coming from a family of many victims.

Much later, after I had developed a working abstract of this book and tentative chapter summaries, I sent copies to them and some other people facing this problem, asking two questions: Would they find this book helpful? What other topics should I include?

The couple responded promptly and soon after, I had lunch with them at their home. In person, they proved to be delightful and interesting people with far different experiences from mine.

It was clear that this is a couple completely devoted to one another. At that point, his symptoms consisted of very mild memory loss, which had not yet even impaired his ability to drive a car alone to his many appointments. He was also able to serve as a volunteer for the Alzheimer's Association, coordinating workshops for newly diagnosed victims and their families.

Both he and his wife had aggressively searched for information about the disease and they were very frank in their assessment of his condition. They regularly attend several meetings and support groups, together and separately. They openly discuss their joint and individual situations with one another and they no doubt have been making decisions regarding the future.

In my thank you note to them for lunch, I wrote:

> "On my way to your house yesterday, I was expecting a conversation in which we would share common experiences with Alzheimer's Disease. Instead, I learned we have had very different experiences and that was highly instructive. For one thing, you two have obviously thoroughly discussed Alzheimer's, your joint and separate reactions and feelings about the disease, how it has affected you now and will in the future, and have developed strategies together to deal with it. Mona and I have never had such a discussion.
> From early 1994 until she was diagnosed in late 2002, although I was sure she had Alzheimer's and said so, we were repeatedly told that we were just dealing with the loss of a memory block for the period of 1990 or so to 1994, which would never be restored, but would never get worse. By the time she was diagnosed, the term Alzheimer's was meaningless to her … she has never used it in connection with herself."

It was then that I realized that I was on my own in this case and that is an awesome responsibility. Nonetheless, I have nearly sixty years of shared memories to draw upon. I believed that I would know when Mona would agree that it was time.

I don't know whether that man's wife has that level of confidence or not. I hope she does. My words to both of them would be those of the legendary Jimmy Durante, "You ain't seen nuttin' yet …" I wish them well.

It is ironic that from the outset, following Mona's diagnosis of Alzheimer's Disease, nearly all of my initial conversations with health care professionals began with them telling me how difficult it was going to be for me to get her into a care facility. For my part, I was interested in how long I could *avoid* doing that. However, I am painfully aware that ultimately, we will have to come to that point.

In mid-2005 Mona's internist, broached the question about what she refers to as Plan B. Plan B is essentially the turning over of the responsibility for Mona's care to someone other than me. More specifically, it is moving her to a Nursing Home or equivalent for her condition.

I suspected, and the doctor admitted that her motivation was principally her perception of and concern for what was happening to me in this process. I have the highest possible level of respect and professional affection for this woman and I deeply appreciated that concern. However, I gently reminded her that she is Mona's Primary Care Physician, not mine.

I asked her if in her professional opinion Mona was suffering in any way because she remained at home with me as the primary Carekeeper. Her answer was no. Nonetheless, I agreed that I should at least begin to think about and develop Plan B.

To some extent, the decision of when to move Mona out of our home is somewhat easier because of the New York State licensing requirements for care facilities. I'm sure that other states have similar regulations.

There are many excellent and very attractive places, euphemistically called "retirement homes", "assisted or enriched living centers", "adult and senior living homes" and "alternatives to Nursing Homes". Many of them advertise that they have "Dementia Units", "Memory Care Programs" and "Alzheimer's Sections", but often it means that the victims are merely restricted to a specific area so they won't wander away. The downside of that is that many victims don't participate in many programs offered by the facility and lead dismal lives. I do not see these facilities being better than having Mona stay at home.

The distinction is in whether these facilities offer skilled nursing services. In New York State, Nursing Homes are, by definition, Skilled Nursing Facilities. Their Alzheimer's, Dementia and Memory Care units are care based, not containment based. There are programs designed for those victims in those units are and they are often very creative.

The requirements for admission to a Nursing Home are higher and come down to answering the following eight cold questions and having an H/C PRI (Hospital/Community Patient Review Instrument) evaluation by a specially trained and certified Registered Nurse:

- Does the person require constant medical monitoring, performed only by a skilled medical professional?

- Does the person require special medications or treatments, administered only by a skilled medical professional?

- Does the person have a tendency to wander if not very closely supervised?

- Does the person sometimes tend to become aggressive and/or violent?

- Can the person move unaided from a sitting position to a standing position?

- Can the person independently dress himself or herself?

- Can the person independently feed himself or herself?

- Can the person independently take care of his or her toileting needs?

Note that there are no questions about the Carekeeper on the list. For the most part, that is as it should be. However, there are also no questions about the level of Dementia including awareness. They deem only the artifacts relevant.

That strikes me as absurd. The combination of the level of Dementia and the non-skilled (in the medical sense) care available are not merely other factors. They are the ultimate factors for consideration, whether positive or negative.

I am sure that there is some kind of weighted scoring for those basic questions and that it is not necessary for all conditions to be present. In mid-2005 when her doctor raised the issue of Plan B, for Mona the answers to all eight questions was no. In reality, however, if this were several years ago, prior to my two hip replacements, I would not be able to handle Mona's care.

If she were to develop either of the first two conditions, the decision would be automatic since I am not considered qualified to provide that level of care and others doing it in our home would not be feasible. Fortunately, her doctor anticipates that neither of those conditions will occur in the near future.

The other six conditions are subjective in their interpretation and in the remedies required to handle them. If one exercises an appropriate level of supervision and stays engaged with the victim, the victim may not wander. Does that mean that they would not under other conditions?

What is the standard for aggressive behavior and where is the line between stubbornness and aggression? For that matter, what is the line between righteous frustration and aggression?

Mona has little or no problems with dressing when I lay out the clothes. I don't need to help her with anything other than coaching her with regard to an efficient sequence. However, if I didn't do that, she would have problems finding and deciding what she should wear. She tends to wear the same things day after day and makes no correlation with weather conditions. That does not represent a yes or no answer to the question posed.

We recently attended a formal wedding. The entrée at the reception was filet mignon served in a creative presentation. Mona had no idea as to how she should deal with it, so I cut about a third of it for her as unobtrusively as possible.

It happened that I had to leave the table for a short while. In my absence, Mona ate all the meat I had cut for her, but had no idea what to do next. I will admit that my menu selections at home are things that are easy for Mona to eat and she has no problem dealing with anything I prepare and serve her, and I would venture to guess, with anything I ordered for her at a restaurant. I can even serve her a salmon steak with just a caution to be careful of bones. The difficulty factor represents a "no" answer to the question about feeding one's self.

As a result, decision-making appears somewhat arbitrary. The easy response is that it depends on the strength and willingness of the Carekeeper. However, that may not be a fair judgment in terms of the welfare of either the victim or that Carekeeper.

In the final analysis, perhaps the decision should have nothing to do with the whims or ability of Carekeeper. Moreover, the Carekeeper may not always be the best judge of how he or she is keeping the proper level of care. The *only* consideration should be that level which is best for the victim. One must always remember that.

Let's consider the next two questions having to do with wandering and violence. Whether dealt with at home or in an institution, the method is the same: control and confine. Certainly that could be handled at home in Mona's case by limiting her freedom to our second floor bedroom, which has a private bath and by installing an outside lock on the door, without imposing too severe burden on me. The question is whether that the best alternative for Mona.

In a care facility the boundaries are often much larger than in our home, allowing access to hallways for walking, rooms for recreation, interaction with other victims and, in some cases, access to controlled, outside areas. Is that a better living environment than I can provide?

There are, however, some important disadvantages, which one must consider. The first is access. There is no Nursing Home next door or down the street. In fact, because of the demand for such facilities, a brief survey indicated that the one of the three facilities considered appropriate for Mona is more than a half hour trip one way from our house. Please note that does not consider the winter weather we experience.

The fifth and sixth questions are, as long as my health remains the same, not severe problems, given our relative size and strength. Besides, Mona is very mobile and shows no signs of slowing down. As far as dressing is concerned, I already have to make the selection of clothing, supervising and coaching the process.

As I proceeded through this analysis, I realized that except for the requirements of full time skilled nursing care, the primary criteria for the decision to move Mona to a Nursing Home should be her personal dignity and not my convenience, sensibilities or pride.

In my current condition and state of health, I believe that I can handle all the tasks on the list of questions about Mona's condition but those first two. The real question requiring an answer is if Mona were making the decision, what criteria would she use. I think she has already provided me with that guidance.

Mealtimes were always special for Mona and still are to some degree, although more and more frequently we eat in silence these days rather than having the animated, stimulating discussions, we once did. Whether they were at home or in a restaurant, these were times for conversation, for kidding, for reminiscing, for enjoying, for both of us. We were equals in that process and it was a time of mutual pleasure, not a mechanical process of the intake of food.

Certainly, I can cut up her food and feed her in silence or in a one-sided dialogue. I am sure that is going to happen before we are through. I can do it because I understand the situation and someone needs to do it. The more salient question is whether she perceives it as an act of devotion and kindness or an embarrassing indignity.

Subsequent to her diagnosis of Wernicke-Korsakoff Syndrome, but well before that of Alzheimer's, Mona developed unrelated Diverticulitis. It was discovered that she had a life-threatening obstruction in her intestine which was about to rupture. This required immediate surgery to remove about twelve inches of her colon. The procedure resulted in Mona having a temporary colostomy. Due to complications from the surgery, she had the colostomy for more than six months.

During that period while Mona was comfortable with going out in public, she was mortified at the thought that I would see her in that condition. For the first time in our marriage, she would lock the bathroom door when she had to deal with the colostomy. It was not Mona's sense of modesty, which was in play; it was her passion for maintaining her dignity.

I believe that the decision determining the point at which I can no longer provide Mona the care she requires, has to do only with her medical condition and maintaining both her persona and her personal dignity. My personal feelings or preferences should not enter into the equation.

My responsibility is that when that time comes, I will have found the appropriate facility and that the transfer will be seamless. I believe that I should not make such a decision under any time pressure.

Therefore, although I did not foresee the need arising for at least another year I began the evaluation and decision process, the first steps in the development of Plan B. That has proven to be an excellent decision.

Mona's Primary Care Physician has told me that we are very fortunate in the Rochester area because there are a large number of excellent Skilled Nursing facilities. With her help and others, I made a list of potential facilities and scheduled visits to each. Since the selection was extensive, I settled on the five that were most highly recommended. As it worked out, four of the five were well within a half hour drive from our home.

I will readily admit that my expectation was that this would be a depressing ordeal. I expected to see long, inadequately lit hallways lined with victims slumped in chairs outside their small and drab rooms doing nothing. I was pleasantly surprised.

Most long established Nursing Homes are faith-based. Although Mona has always been a practicing Catholic, I did not consider that a primary requirement, since for her those distinctions have clearly become irrelevant in this instance. Therefore, of the five I selected, one was Baptist affiliated, one Jewish, one non-denominational and the other two Catholic oriented.

The consensus among those who had advised me was that the front-runner would be the Jewish Home, since that had been the standard for a number of years. It is also the easiest to get to from our house. The fact is that I was impressed with all five and would have few qualms if Mona spent the rest of her days in any one of them.

My tour was instructive, however, because although there were significant differences between them, none stood far above the rest. Conversely, none was demonstrably lacking. I think that it would be useful to discuss what I found from the perspective of what one should look for and find.

It was interesting that all five realized that they were doing the job well. I was up front on each visit, explaining that I was looking at five places and identifying them. The universal response was that I was doing the right thing and that I had chosen the top five in the area. It was readily apparent that they were well aware of what the others were doing and, although each had a waiting list, they are all very competitive without criticizing anyone.

One had a very innovative environmental approach and the other four were trying to emulate it, were in the process of doing so, or were planning a total renovation to improve on it. This approach is unique in the area and perhaps in the state. At least three of the remaining four told of specific plans to implement that approach at least partially.

They divided the entire facility divided into twenty self-contained "communities" of nine to twelve residents. By the simple expedient of re-orienting the aspect ratio of rooms to be parallel to the external wall of the wing instead of perpendicular, they opened the previously conventional center hallway into an area of great creative potential. The difference was dramatic.

There is a mix of single and double rooms and they gave the impression of being larger than others I had seen, with good storage and space for a reclining chair and other furniture. The double rooms afford privacy by the use of fixed two-sided entertainment units as well as the usual curtain dividing them. Each room had a private lavatory.

The Nursing Station was now in the center of the action, along with the main activity and dining areas, greatly facilitating supervision. Two "communities" share one Registered Nurse and two Aides staff each community during the day and evening, with one on duty overnight.

In addition to the central open area, there was also a pleasant and comfortable "quiet area" defined by walls with tastefully designed multi-paned windows so it didn't feel like an observation room. When requested this space is scheduled for family visits and even private meals.

Those family meals can be prepared in fully equipped, very functional and spacious kitchens in each "community" from which they serve the meals from a central kitchen. There are stocked cupboards and a refrigerator. Snacks can be prepared throughout the day and night.

All of the facilities had separate areas for the care of advanced stage Alzheimer's victims. I did not feel it was necessary to visit those areas based on the level of care I had observed.

Although this was clearly the standard, which the four other facilities I visited emulated with varying levels of success. The least successful one has embarked on an extensive two-year renovation program and I would suspect that when it is complete, it would be the new standard. Unfortunately, Mona having to endure the renovation process probably takes that facility out of consideration until it is completed.

All five had substantial waiting lists but they also had policies of no obligation, no deposit applications. In some cases, the application remains inactive until the family notifies them to activate it. One or two however, offer an applicant accommodation when they reach the top of the list when they have a one-time right of refusal before going inactive.

There is a very troubling downside to this course of action. Mona would have to give up the care of her Primary Care Physician. She tells me that while she would like to continue to provide that care, each of the facilities under consideration has staff doctors and do not grant privileges to outsiders.

I could understand that position if Mona were unable to go to the doctor's office. I do not understand that position, as long as I am able to take her there. I planned to pursue the possibility of negotiating some kind of compromise.

This process had been very instructive for me and I decided that I would make applications for Mona for the four facilities, which were not planning massive renovations in the short term. Submission of these applications requires the completion of the Hospital/Community Patient Review Instrument (H/C PRI), which I mentioned early. Plan B was underway and I needed to see how close Mona was to qualifying for Skilled Nursing Care.

I must take a point of personal privilege on this blatant example of one of the bureaucratic absurdities in our health care system. Despite its nearly comical simplicity and lack of sophistication, which is within the capabilities of someone with an eighth grade education, a specially certified, registered nurse must complete the PRI. As a result, the time between my request that the survey be done and the arrival of a "qualified" person to do it, was four months.

That is ridiculous enough, but evaluating the survey took another month. That is not the end of the absurdity. The survey is only valid for three months. To stay current, one must request the renewal at the same time as the initial survey and a second renewal a month before they do the first renewal.

Even the need for frequent renewal is ridiculous. The stated purpose is to safeguard against the use of the PRI by a victim who no longer qualifies for Nursing Home care. Apparently, no one has told them that Alzheimer's is incurable.

I should add that there is a substantial fee for completing the PRI. What a surprise.

The nurse completed the survey without talking with Mona or even asking a question that would shed any light on her condition. In fact, Mona was not present during the interview.

Ironically, the initial PRI score did not indicate that Mona required Nursing Home care. However, a week or so before the PRI, the doctor and nurses conducting the clinical trial in which Mona participated for two years said that based on her standard test scores, if they didn't know her, they would have concluded that she was in bed, in a fetal position at some Nursing Home.

I might conclude that the discrepancy between the two analyses was so that the people doing the PRI could collect for at least one more survey. I won't draw that conclusion because I don't want to appear cynical.

At Mona's final appointment in the clinical study, the doctor and the principal nurse involved asked me what I was planning to do regarding Mona and when. My response was that I would continue to do what I am doing as long as it is in Mona's best interest.

They both said that they thought the results of my approach, while somewhat unconventional, were remarkable in the sense that she remains nearly fully functional and essentially independent, while being severely afflicted.

Recently, I had a conversation with a woman who has been a friend of Mona's for more than forty years and she had asked how Mona was. They don't see each other much more than occasionally at church, but just a couple weeks ago they had a brief conversation.

When I mentioned Mona and Alzheimer's in the same sentence, she was shocked. I told her that she must be the only person in Pittsford who didn't know. However, that is an example of how functional Mona *appears* to be as compared to the stark reality of the actual situation.

When the doctor pressed me on when I would make the decision to turn Mona's care over to someone else, I said that I would try to do it between the time when I desperately wanted her to stay and when I desperately wanted her to go. I would not like to spend the rest of my life regretting that I had missed that window.

AFTERWORD

▼

I completed the manuscript for this book in early summer of 2006, when proof reading and a final edit began. Ironically, during the same period several significant changes occurred in Mona's situation. The speed with which they moved resulted in a reciprocal slowing of the completion of the book.

Rather than to do an extensive rewrite of Chapter Eleven I decided that it was more appropriate to handle those changes and their consequences in an "Afterword". I believe that was a good decision if only as an illustration and affirmation of the old cliché from Robert Burns about "the best laid plans of mice and men ..."

Mona had a scheduled three-month check-up with her Primary Care Physician in early June and since our daughter Maryellen happened to be in town, she went along. During the appointment, I reported the following changes in Mona during the prior three months:

- She had two obvious, though very minor instances, which were possibly instances of wandering.

- She had shown new levels of confrontation, bordering on aggressive behavior, once with the Home Health Care Aide and twice with me.

- She was having increased episodes of bowel incontinence, approaching several times per week.

- She was having increased difficulty with dressing.

- She was increasingly incapable of intelligible conversation, sometimes managing it even less than once a day.

I knew that this was a significant level of change in just three months. The doctor listened intently, then looked me straight in the eye and said simply, "It is time for Plan B".

We had been in this project together much too long for a ceremonial argument. I replied, "I know".

I immediately began one final survey of Skilled Nursing Facilities on my own. A couple of weeks later, one of our granddaughters and her husband came over from Boston at my request to do an independent assessment. I scheduled their appointments, but did not accompany them on their visits so that I would not influence their thinking.

They had been extraordinarily well prepared for their task, with pages of questions for each location and lists of criteria by which they would make their judgments. We discussed their findings over dinner that night.

We ranked the same facility fourth and I decided against applying there. Their ranking of the top three varied slightly from mine, principally because one of the facilities had an adjacent independent living building with one-bedroom efficiency apartments, which they liked. I had previously decided that was irrelevant and they were not aware that I felt that way.

By early July, I submitted the applications with supporting documentation to the top three and we had an updated PRI done. It showed that Mona clearly qualified for Skilled Nursing Care.

Each of the facilities said that the typical waiting period was three months. I assumed incorrectly that it was unlikely that they were all on the same cycle; that it was unlikely that the three month waiting period was consistently exceeded; and with three applications active an acceptance was likely to come in as little as two months and would not exceed four.

So much for the statistical approach, but based on that faulty logic I decided that consistent with my intention to not stay in the house after Mona moved and cognizant of the impending reality of winter I should be ready to move as early September 1, which would allow for disposing of the house before any serious snowfall. However, I did not mount any particular effort to make that happen.

Nonetheless, early one Sunday morning on my way back from the store with breakfast fixings, I noticed a sign at the entrance of a street I had never seen in the previous forty-two years. On a whim, I turned in. I found an attractive apartment complex that I didn't know existed, although it is less than four miles from our house.

I looked at a couple of apartments the next day and decided that one of them satisfied every requirement I could imagine. I signed a lease, effective September 1. I cannot emphasize sufficiently the salutary effect that action had. I had effectively disconnected my expected future from the uncertainty of Mona's.

Subsequent to Mona's appointment with her doctor in early June, most of the symptoms I had reported had continued to develop and intensify. Concurrently, whether because of her increasing difficulty in carrying on a cogent conversation or not, Mona seemed to withdraw steadily. She became more docile and serene, but communication between us essentially stopped and reduced to looks of appreciation when I helped her dress, performed simple tasks for her or served her meals.

I have long been a believer in the "squeaky wheel theory" and conducted a campaign of gentle pressure on the three skilled nursing facilities. Without fail, every other Friday, I called the Directors of Admission at each. Although they assured me that they welcomed my call, I sensed that they knew how to make me stop and were more likely than not to try to make that happen.

In the case of one of these facilities, during a period some fifteen years earlier I had known the CEO reasonably well and several members of her Board, including her brother even better. None of them was any longer active, but the Pastor of our parish was. In addition, this facility also operated the Day Care Center Mona had attended for three years. I contacted all of them to plead Mona's case and the Day Care Center Director offered to act as an advocate. The others were less responsive.

At the beginning of the third month, I added another kind of pressure. I did some research and found the names of the Medical Directors at each facility. I then contacted Mona's Primary Care Physician and asked her to make a peer contact with each of them on Mona's behalf. She readily agreed to do that.

I am not sure which of these tactics, if any had an effect. However, on October 24, just four days after I had a "no change" response from each of the three, I had a call from The Friendly Home, offering Mona a room. They gave me 24 hours to accept or reject the offer and move her in. I successfully negotiated an extension to 36 hours and conditionally accepted the offer, contingent on inspecting the room offered.

Ironically, just five days earlier our daughter learned that she had breast cancer and was facing surgery, chemotherapy and radiation. Not only did that significantly affect my mental and emotional state of mind, but our plan had been that when Mona was accepted Maryellen would fly in to help me make that happen. One final element of "the ultimate do-it-yourself project".

Fortunately, Maryellen's surgery exactly one week after the call from The Friendly Home went smoothly. As I write this, she has completed her six chemo treatments and six weeks of daily radiation. After another check up, her doctor declared her free of cancer and the prognosis is encouraging.

The room offered Mona was about as good as anyone could anticipate. All of the rooms are double occupancy but hers was a corner room at the end of the hall, which meant that it was slightly larger than the others were and had the additional benefit of large windows on two walls.

I accepted it on the spot. Twenty-four hours later, Mona and I headed from our house to The Friendly Home, two hastily packed suitcases in the back seat. Mona accepted all this without questioning.

When we arrived at our destination, Mona got out of the car without incident. I left her bags in the car.

The plan was that I would ask the Receptionist to inform the Social Worker that we had arrived and we headed for to the room. The Social Worker would join us there.

The route to her room was down a pleasant corridor past the main dining room, a small activities room, a gift shop and a small snack bar. On one side of the corridor were windows looking out onto a large, enclosed garden patio. On the other side, there was an art exhibit by a local artist.

Mona was like an excited child, marveling at how nice everything looked. At the end of the corridor, we took an elevator up one floor where I punched in an access code on a keypad to open the door to the main corridor of the Dementia Unit.

The Nurse Supervisor was there to greet us and take us down to Mona's room. She could see into it before we reached it and Mona said, "Oh, look how pretty that room is!" Then she saw her name on the door and that really pleased her.

She was eagerly looking around when the Social Worker arrived. After introducing herself to Mona, she asked if she would like to see the activities room and the dining room. Mona said, "Sure!"

It was a cold day and Mona was wearing a winter down jacket. I said I'd take her coat and moved close to unzip it. My face was less than a foot from hers. I looked her straight in the eye and said, "This is where you live now".

She looked a little surprised and asked "Forever?" I replied, "Yes, forever".

After a slight pause, Mona said "Wow! That's great!" Off she went with the Nurse.

Later I realized that the conversation I had with Mona from our arrival until that moment, was the most lucid in many months. Somehow, that helped me a great deal.

The Social Worker urged me to leave at that point and except for bringing in Mona's suitcases from the car, not to see her for at least twenty-four hours. That was a strange experience.

Earlier I mentioned that there were three Skilled Nursing Facilities under consideration, Fairport Baptist Home, Friendly Home and St. Ann's Home. In our evaluation of the three, although my granddaughter and her husband and I agreed that all three facilities were very acceptable there was a discrepancy in our ranking.

I had ranked them Fairport Baptist, St. Ann's and Friendly Home. I chose Fairport Baptist as first because of their innovative layout of facilities. Although St. Ann's was the farthest away and Friendly Home the closest, I ranked St. Ann's slightly higher because it was Catholic and Friendly Home is non-denominational.

Megan and Dave ranked the three in exactly the reverse order. They preferred Friendly Home because it has that adjacent building with apartments for spouses of patients, which did not interest me at all.

In retrospect, I am not sure whether my preference for the innovative layout of Fairport Baptist is of any consequence to the resident although it seems very attractive to their relatives. The ranking of St. Ann's as preferable since it is Catholic, although significantly farther away has also been subject to a degree of re-evaluation.

Mona and I are both lifelong, practicing Catholics and our religion is a source of strength as well as comfort. If Mona's disease were physical rather than mental, that would become very high priority. For the Alzheimer's victim that is probably not a relevant factor. Nonetheless, not a week goes by that Mona is not visited by a representative of our parish or a nearby sister parish just down the street from The Friendly Home.

I have become very impressed with the non-profit, non-denominational Friendly Home. Founded in 1849, it is recognized as one of the premier skilled nursing facilities in the area. I have concluded that excellence of care is the critical consideration and I believe that Mona is in the best possible environment.

Since she has been there, I have discovered something I did not know about Alzheimer's Disease. The unit she is in has twenty-two "guests". Currently the ratio of women to men is seven to one. I asked the nurse the other day if that was unusual. She said that in her twenty years in the unit the majority has always been heavily women.

In all the reading I have done, I had never come across anything that would indicate the large disparity. Some more specific research I did recently turned up information that adjusted for age, seven of ten Alzheimer's victims are women and that there has been research begun to see if the cause might be hormonal.

I recently attended my 55th college reunion, where I learned of three classmates newly diagnosed with Alzheimer's. When we graduated, men outnumbered women in our class by four to one. Two of the three new cases were women.

In accordance with my plan, sixteen days after Mona moved to The Friendly Home, with the essential assistance of our son from California, his brother, brother's wife and daughters, two Boston based granddaughters and their spouses, I moved into the apartment I had leased earlier. It is 3.3 miles from The Friendly Home.

As I write this, Mona has lived at The Friendly Home for eight months and I have lived in my apartment for seven. I visit Mona nearly every day. She is pleased to see me arrive and content to see me go. There is serenity about her and she seems happy.

One day, she was sitting in the lounge area of the unit with perhaps ten or twelve of the other residents. She saw me approaching and raised her hand high in the gesture we have used for years on such occasions. Then she began to clap. Her colleagues joined in and I entered the area to an ovation, albeit a sitting ovation, but an ovation nonetheless.

Shortly after Mona moved into The Friendly Home and I moved into my apartment, I found myself in what I described in an e-mail to my closest friend as a "funk". Her response was:

> "I don't think you are in a funk. I think your body is reacting to all that's been going on for years and especially the last few months. Think about it…. Mona and your care for her, then her move and no more care for her, your move and all that involved with what to keep/what to throw, deciding what to do with the house and the emotions involved with having lived there for so many years, the holidays being the first ones not in your home and without Mona there, Maryellen's emotional and frightening crisis … get the picture? You have to give yourself time to adjust and readjust, realign, reevaluate, accept and proceed. It will take time and you need to give in to your body's needs of rest, recuperation, relaxation and rejuvenation. It will happen … sermon over.
> The requirement to manage two lives in great detail is VERY strenuous/stressful! You'll get your rhythm and groove back … it will just take some time and you need to allow yourself that time. Don't be too hard on yourself with needing to set priorities. You're not a person who wastes time … this IS a time for yourself … waste some time if it feels good! You've earned it!"

She was correct. I soon began to make the readjustment. I also reached a level of contentment and strangely felt a sense of accomplishment and pride. I did the best I could.

978-0-595-49075-2
0-595-49075-1

Printed in the United States
204805BV00002B/268-351/P